Praise for *Befriending the North Wind*

Weaving insights from philosophy, theology, anthropology, developmental psychology, and pediatrics into a nuanced account of the moral agency of children, Robyn Boeré has authored a book of exceptional wisdom and sensitivity. In paying attention to what dying children actually say and do rather than forcing upon them the rickety bioethical principles of a society that fears death and worships autonomy, Boeré shows what children can teach adults about being interdependent creatures made in God's image. As a pediatrician and parent, I highly recommend *Befriending the North Wind* to anyone who cares about the moral and spiritual lives of children.

—Brian Volck, MD, MFA, MAT, coauthor of *Reclaiming the Body: Christians and the Faithful Use of Modern Medicine* and author of *Attending Others: A Doctor's Education in Bodies and Words*

I can think of no higher praise for Robyn Boeré's *Befriending the North Wind* than to say it is a lovely book, not simply because of the effortlessness with which the author writes about the stories of George McDonald, but also because of the opportunity she affords readers to change the way they see and speak about life and death, not just of children but also of themselves. By drawing on the stories of Jesus and children in the Gospels and Saint Paul's use of familial metaphors to describe the relationship of the baptized to the triune God, Boeré makes the daring claim that "childness is humanness." Recognizing the moral agency of children opens the possibility of seeing them not simply as capable of shaping their own living and dying, but as exemplars of dying well. Insofar as the goal of Christian discipleship is to live as a child of God, she concludes, "we should all die as children."

—Joel James Shuman, professor of theology, King's College, Wilkes-Barre, Pennsylvania

Befriending
the
North Wind

Befriending
the
North Wind

Children, Moral Agency, and the Good Death

Robyn Boeré

FORTRESS PRESS
MINNEAPOLIS

BEFRIENDING THE NORTH WIND
Children, Moral Agency, and the Good Death

Library of Congress Cataloging-in-Publication Data

Names: Boeré, Robyn, author.
Title: Befriending the North Wind : children, moral agency, and the good
    death / Robyn Boeré.
Description: Minneapolis : Fortress Press, [2023] | Includes
    bibliographical references and index.
Identifiers: LCCN 2023016394 (print) | LCCN 2023016395 (ebook) | ISBN
    9781506481838 (paperback) | ISBN 9781506481845 (ebook)
Subjects: LCSH: Terminally ill children--Care--Moral and ethical aspects. |
    Terminal care--Moral and ethical aspects. | Terminal care--Religious
    aspects--Christianity. | Children and death--Religious
    aspects--Christianity.
Classification: LCC RJ249 .B64 2023 (print) | LCC RJ249 (ebook) | DDC
    362.19892/005--dc23/eng/20230601
LC record available at https://lccn.loc.gov/2023016394
LC ebook record available at https://lccn.loc.gov/2023016395

Cover design: Kristin Miller

Cover image: Pine Tree in the Wind—stock image ©CSA-Printstock |
Getty Images

Print ISBN: 978-1-5064-8183-8
eBook ISBN: 978-1-5064-8184-5

To AMB, who shared with me the joys and pains
of childhood from our earliest moments,
and to RER, who has never lost her childlike wonder.
Thank you.

The combination of assets and liabilities that an adult brings to a philosophical encounter with a child makes for a very special relationship. The adult has a better command of the language than the child and, latently at least, a truer command of the concepts expressed in the language. It is the child, however, who has fresh eyes and ears for perplexity and incongruity. Children also have, typically, a degree of candor and spontaneity that is hard for the adult to match. Because each party has something important to contribute, the inquiry can easily become a genuinely joint venture, something otherwise quite rare between adults and children. Some adults are not prepared to face a child stripped of the automatic presumption of adults' superiority in knowledge and experience.

—Gareth Matthews

When I became a man I put away childish things, including the fear of childishness and the desire to be very grown up.

—C. S. Lewis

Truly I tell you, anyone who will not receive the kingdom of God like a little child will never enter it.

—Mark 10:15

Contents

Introduction

Barely Seen, Rarely Heard

Death meets us all. Nothing in nature escapes its veiled countenance. All sowing gives way to reaping. But death's embrace often feels unnatural, especially when it visits a child. A moral dissonance arises from such visitations. The promise, newness, and hope for the future symbolized in youth and youth's maturation are violated by death's indifference. And it is not only we moderns—equipped as we are with cutting-edge medicine, technology, and expertise—who feel this special dread. Past generations, who endured much higher levels of child mortality, felt death's sting no less sharply.

The death of a child horrifies. It calls the whole world into question. It invites us to doubt our highest notions: purpose, justice, God, and the meaning of human life. We recoil at its mention, yet certain images prevent us from averting our gaze. Images of dead or dying children—the Syrian boy washed up on the shores of an Italian beach; Charlie Gard lying intubated on a hospital bed—demand our attention in ways that challenge us to change our behavior, but too often result in despair's inaction. Most of the time the topic of dying children is studiously avoided. When dying children do impose themselves on our notice, they are painted as victims, innocent of both blame and agency, the ideal of passivity in the face of suffering. Children die secluded in homes and hospitals, allowing society to carry on as though it were not happening. To overcome our avoidance and the moral cowardice that funds it, we must find models that help us approach this subject in a more constructive way.

Child death is the central theme of George MacDonald's book *At the Back of the North Wind*. It tells the story of Diamond, the young son of a coachman, who first meets North Wind when she is blowing through a little hole in the wall of his bedroom.[1] In the months that follow, she takes Diamond on many adventures, whisking him through the rooftops of London fulfilling her tasks—tasks that include the sinking of a large vessel, for one of North Wind's other names is Death. Despite his fear of the destruction waged by North Wind, Diamond learns to trust her and gradually hears from her about the existence of the world "at her back." The connection between death and North Wind is heightened when Diamond's visit to the world at her back is preceded by his mother's concern that he is getting ill; when he returns from that world, he wakes to find he has been very ill indeed. Not much about the world at the back of North Wind is explicitly depicted; much like the ecstatic experience of the beatific vision, it can only be remembered in fragments and is almost impossible for Diamond to describe. Many of Diamond's experiences with North Wind—the feeling of cold, fear, and discomfort, losing track of time in sickness—will be familiar to children who have experienced serious illness. After his recovery, he almost forgets his friend North Wind, though never completely, and he is changed by his friendship with her. After many other adventures and the telling of many fairy tales and poems, Diamond goes permanently to the back of the North Wind. That is, he dies.

Contemporary readers may balk at the notion that death can be befriended. In a culture that glorifies health and youth, the death of a child stands counter to all our notions of what childhood should be. How, then, is it possible to befriend such a horror, to willingly go to the back of the North Wind? Readers today may also be concerned about the juxtaposition of worldly suffering and otherworldly reward. It seems to suggest that childhood suffering is made right by the promise of heavenly bliss. But MacDonald never suggests this; he never denies the goodness of this life, only that the next is even better. And there are aspects of the story we ought to criticize, like the accepted classism and gender relationships of the Victorian age (though this too MacDonald rebukes). Like all stories, it is a product of its time. But like all good stories, it can awaken in each generation new ways of seeing the world. What is remarkable about this book, and should provoke conflict in contemporary readers, is how Diamond is transformed through his journeys with North Wind. After his first visit to the world "at her back," he is less talkative. He is more empathetic to the suffering of others. He invents nonsense poetry. He can recognize in the faces of others those who have also visited the world at North Wind's back. In contrast to the contemporary commitment to the view that suffering, dying, and death are inherently meaningless, *At the Back of the North Wind* suggests that dying can be personally and morally transformative.

At the Back of the North Wind, and MacDonald's wider fairy-tale corpus, both imaginatively evoke and theologically shape many of the themes of this book: creative reasoning, multiplicity of meaning, childlike moral agency, and eternal childhood. MacDonald was writing in a cultural context struggling, like us, with new questions about the meaning of childhood. MacDonald, who himself lost three of his thirteen children to illness, was concerned with problems that still present a challenge to us today, and in ways that are pressing in pediatric palliative medicine: the primacy of cold analytic (adult male, for MacDonald) reasoning, the loss of faith in the afterlife, a romanticized view of childhood. His stories are not a manual for us today, but they do serve to spark our imagination to consider how the truths expressed in these stories can be made real to us now. These truths, that we are all children of God, and that there is real hope in the resurrection, are foundational to my project. This does not erase the suffering of the present. It does not make child death, or any death, somehow "okay." But there is real hope in the way that death has been transformed from the end of life to a gateway to eternal life.[2] Through fairy tale, we can imaginatively explore how that might be, and learn to hold onto what we know in faith to be true even when, confronted with tragedy in our lives, it feels furthest from real.

To be inspired by stories seems to me appropriate for this book, which will consider the strengths children bring to moral inquiry, especially at the end of life, and how they, along with those around them, can prepare for death. Children are powerful reminders of the necessity of story in the human life. As Canadian anthropologist Hugh Brody says, "The human mind depends on speaking and listening, hearing and telling stories. If there is silence, then there is much about who we are that we cannot know. Silence in the home can leave a void in a child."[3] Silence at the deathbed can do the same. One of the reasons we find the death of children so tragic is that we worry they do not have the capacity to create a narrative that gives meaning to their lives.[4] This concern not only overlooks the incredible capacities that children do have, but also ignores the role of *shared* stories, of telling stories to children, and of encouraging them to tell stories. Children are able to learn and explore who they are through story. It should come as no surprise, then, that fairy tales and fantasy stories are one of the main vehicles for discussing death.[5]

Those of us living in modern industrialized nations with widespread sanitation, vaccination programs, selective abortions, and public health support are among the first few generations in human history who have not confronted child death as a commonplace occurrence. Childhood mortality, estimated to have been as high as 50 percent in ancient and medieval Europe, is now statistically rare. There is something almost miraculous about the way in which infant and child mortality has declined in the past 200 years in industrialized countries. For adults in modern Europe, North America, and parts of Asia, Africa, and South America, this decline means that only a small minority of us have lost a sibling or child, and few of us will have witnessed a child's death. Because of this transformation, childhood, which has always to some extent represented hope and possibility, has taken on a more simplistic meaning: a passing stage of life on the way to "real life." The purpose of childhood is to prepare for the real life of adulthood. The work of childhood is to grow up. When children today are sick or die, it happens far from public view—glimpsed darkly through TV, telethons, and fundraising campaigns. When child death imposes itself more directly, it results in moral panic.

Moral panic leads to hasty solutions. And hasty solutions tend to exacerbate problems. In medical ethics, we see this impulse in a few ways: First, in the growing enthusiasm for euthanasia, and pushes for euthanasia to be extended by right to ever younger cohorts of people. Child euthanasia is now legal in Belgium and the Netherlands, and there is pressure in Canada to follow suit. This push is often part of a larger trend of extending decision-making rights wholesale to younger and younger citizens. Conversely, a strong push exists in some areas for the opposite—that is, for guaranteeing so-called family privacy (which affords parents total autonomy for decisions). Both trends simplify the morally fraught questions of medical decision-making and care for children, both in general and at the end of life. This oversimplification is compounded by a tendency in medical ethics to adjust individualistic, adult-driven models of rights and agency to suit the needs of children, rather than to rethink decision-making wholesale. Less tangible but equally important is the pervasive notion that childhood suffering is anathema and must be eliminated at all costs. Rarely does the scholarly conversation widen to consider the role that our views of childhood, moral agency, and death play in directing our intuitions, reasoning, and public policy. Child death and suffering lead us to seek an immediate response, without doing the difficult work of overcoming our inadequate ideas.

Instead of seeking quick fixes, we must face important questions about (1) who children are, (2) how we treat them, (3) what we owe them, and (4) how to include them. Our reasoning is only as good as the truth of its premises. If we hold mistaken beliefs about children, their moral agency, their humanity, and their deaths, we will misconstrue ethical situations involving children and only exacerbate the harm done to them. Our choices are limited by the stories we tell, and the stories we tell about children in contemporary Western culture have serious limitations and sometimes contain outright errors. To understand a child, we must look beyond the realm of medicine and address questions of theology. We must focus attention on the central subject of pediatric ethics: the child.

✳✳✳

Today, discussions of child death and illness happen almost exclusively within the medical system, in pediatric hospitals and hospices. This monopoly is not unique to pediatric care. The last century has seen a seismic shift in the locations where people die and, relatedly, in the methods and aims of end-of-life care. This change in location is about more than the proliferation of hospital systems and care centers; it is a movement of cultural space. For modern culture, death is a *medical* problem, and so people die in the places where medicine is practiced.

But for much of history, people died at home, sometimes in the same bed in which they were born. Death was—and not untroublingly so—part of everyday life. One of the shocking elements of reading *At the Back of the North Wind* is that physicians and hospitals are almost entirely absent. Care for the dying person was largely the task of family members (though hospices of various kinds have existed for centuries). In rituals like the medieval *ars moriendi* and in the litanies of many prayer books, we witness a deathly anxiety quite different from our own, one reflected in the recurrent petitions that one will not die suddenly and unprepared. It is not death's mere visitation that elicits fear and warrants divine entreaty, but rather its furtive arrival. The Christian pilgrim prayed to be made ready for death's advent and to be spared the terror of that visitor showing up unannounced.

Medicalization changes the stories we tell ourselves about death and dying. In the medical story, death is the enemy against whom we wage war, never a friend whose arrival we anticipate. The dying process is not preparatory or transformative, but inherently meaningless. Cures should always be sought. Suffering is never instructive and should be avoided as the greatest of evils. Dying is an event of the physical body, not a journey of the soul.

The medicalization of death should be appreciated for the massive improvement in symptom management and pain relief at the end of life. It has more recently also meant increased access to therapists, chaplains, and other professionals trained to help people cope with the spiritual, emotional, and psychological aspects of dying. The latter has happened especially through the pushback of palliative and hospice care, which have questioned the primacy of "cure" in medicine. But the medicalization of death has also redefined death itself. One theologian goes so far as to say the medicalization of dying "prematurely alienate[s] people from their own bodies, from their communities, and from God."[6] Views of death have been affected by medicine's inability to accept death. For child death, cultural inability to accept that children die meets this medical rejection of death to create an especially potent mix. Opposite the otherwise strong disparity in medical studies involving children, 60 percent of children participate in clinical trials for novel therapies compared with 2 percent of adults.[7] Whereas adults are often referred to palliative care with months or years to live, pediatric palliative referrals and do not resuscitate (DNR) discussions frequently happen late in the disease's trajectory, often only hours or days before a child dies.[8]

This premature alienation from self and community has an especially profound effect on children. Dying children often feel ignored, overlooked, and unable to exercise their agency to ameliorate their situation (or even participate in defining what their situation is). Hospitals are notoriously difficult places for children to express their experiences and act on their own behalf. We know so little about how children themselves view the hospital, their bodies, their illness, their prognosis, and their priorities. The small sample size for study is both a blessing in that child death is now comparatively rare, but concerning because we are in the dark about the challenges facing children with life-limiting illness. One researcher goes so far as to say that the price for the decrease in child mortality is paid by seriously ill children, their parents, and medical staff.[9] The fewer children who die, the easier it is for us to sustain the illusion that children don't die at all. It also allows the mistaken idea to flourish that shielding children from any knowledge of death is both possible and laudable.

This mistake and the illusion that sustains it contribute to the understandable concern families have regarding talking about death or allowing researchers to study children who are dying. We worry that asking children to talk about their experiences will compound their suffering, that mentioning pain and death will in some way make them finally real. Parents have a deep desire to protect their children from unnecessary burdens. And while such intent is right, the resulting actions ignore the fact that children want to talk about their experiences, want to communicate their knowledge about their disease and prognosis, and want to ask questions about death. Children initiate conversations about death with their families; it is only when families and physicians refuse to engage that children become silent. One physician recalls how deep this silencing can go: When a teenage girl in his care found her attempts to talk about death rebuffed, she stopped talking altogether in her final few months of life.[10]

When we judge the topic of death too painful, too difficult, and too intellectually demanding for children, it is dying children who suffer most. This lack of communication stems from the refusal of parents and other caregivers to admit to themselves the truth about disease progression. This refusal has several consequences. Children are subjected to unrealistic treatment decisions which are often associated with significant physical suffering. Their spiritual and emotional needs are not met (research shows they frequently hide their knowledge of their prognosis as an act of care for those around them). But it is also those around the dying child who suffer. Many families express regret that they did not talk about dying with their child. This silence also contributes to the suffering of siblings, many of whom feel a complex mix of emotions including guilt and sorrow. Finally, silence eliminates the chance for children to tell stories about their own death that can make their experiences meaningful and, in turn, teach the living what it means to die well.

Philosopher Gareth Matthews argues that issues specific to children are ignored because "claims about childhood tend to fall into the category of the obvious."[11] Adults think we know what children want because we deem their wants obvious. As "obvious," there is nothing to gain from close study. Take, for example, assumptions about children's preferred place of death. Many policy documents claim that children want to die at home, and advocates strongly argue for that opportunity to be provided. But the claim itself is not supported by any meaningful evidence. Instead, it relies on a mix of assumptions and data extrapolated from surveying adults. A systematic review of the literature on preferred place of death found only nine studies specifically about place-of-death preferences among children and young people. Of these, most only interviewed parents, primarily mothers. Even these limited studies demonstrated that what was already taken as obvious—that children wish to die at home—is, from the perspective of parents, not necessarily true. But neither the studies nor the assumptions they affirm necessarily reflect what children want. We simply do not know what children want because no study has asked them.[12]

As the medicalization of death overdetermines death's meaning, it obscures nonmedical meaning and nonmedical concerns at the end of life. A dying child is a whole person. Their concerns at the end of life are as varied and personal as those of adults. The setting of child death can prompt us to think predominantly of the medical, but while we may be concerned most about whether the current treatment is working, a child may be most concerned about the equitable division of her Lego collection among her siblings and friends. Children may want to decide how to dispose of their possessions, and frequently have strong views on this. Many children want to be involved in planning their funerals. Other decisions include deciding the preferred location of death, which is not solely a medical decision. A child may also want to decide who should be there when they are dying, and whether to receive the sacraments or other rituals of their faith.

The ability of children to participate in their end-of-life care is limited not only by cultural and parental views, but by the moral systems at work in medicine. Typical models of medical decision-making fail children in need. Recent studies have highlighted the discrepancy between children's desire to participate and their opportunities for doing so. Impediments to children's participation come to a head in the intractable cases of conflict between family members, or between families and the health-care team responsible for care plans. Families do not always act in the best interest of their children. And the intellectual, social, and cultural biases of care providers lead to drastically different patterns of care depending on the race, gender, and social status of the child.

At its philosophical root, autonomy shapes our cultural ideas of decision-making. Autonomy is not value-neutral but contains normative ideas about what it means to be human and to act in the human world. The lives of children are characterized by a culture in which autonomy shapes what it means to be rational and to make decisions. It is on this basis that the stark divide between children and adults is culturally predicated. Autonomy is, in most Western countries, *the* standard of participation in moral realms and social spaces. It is the bedrock of moral medicine. With its images of the rugged individualist, rational, maximizing chooser, it has been a strong contributor to the notion that children are at best proto-moral, because true morality relies on the actualization of selective rational capacities.

Autonomy is one of Childress and Beauchamp's four principles of bioethics, first articulated in their seminal 1979 book. It is autonomy, in their definition, that allows for meaningful choices. Pediatric bioethics has not differed significantly from this approach, except that it is common for pediatric bioethics to rearrange or increase the number of principles in light of the complexities involved in making medical decisions for children. Child medical ethics gives primacy of place to beneficence (one of the other principles). It is families, generally, who are granted the autonomy to decide what is in the best interest of their children and thus define beneficence. The dominance of autonomy is tied to a procedural account of moral decision-making; it is the fact that the decision is "mine" that makes it moral. In the case of children, then, there is little guidance: They cannot make decisions that are properly "theirs" because they lack the deliberative capacity that comes only with adulthood (or so the story goes).

In theory, medical decision-making models hold to a decision-specific account of capacity, meaning that only enough capacity for a given decision is needed, rather than meeting a general criterion. For example, while the decision about in which arm to receive a vaccine jab could be made by almost anyone, the decision to start or end chemotherapy is far more complex. But the reality is that most children are presumed to be generally incapable. Many capacity-based models assert that children lack the necessary capacities for meaningful input. But in many individual decisions, the only difference between an adult and a child is that the adult is presumed to have capacity (and must prove otherwise by some mad act), while the child is presumed to lack it and must prove otherwise, usually in clear, literal language. In addition, because capacity-based models are highly individualistic, attention is generally given only to what children can achieve on their own. Of course, many families do include children in decisions, but in most places, this is based on their willingness rather than an inherent right of the child.

Astonishingly, many pediatric ethics handbooks do not mention involving children in contentious care decisions. In Carter, Levetown, and Friebert's *Palliative Care for Infants, Children, and Adolescents: A Practical Handbook*, there are two case studies presented involving children who are old enough to speak and capable of interaction—one involving whether a seven-year-old with leukemia should be transferred to a hospice, and another case involving a ten-year-old with a brain tumor—but no mention is made in either case of the children's opinions, values, thoughts, desires, wishes, or their experience of illness, hospitalization, or treatment. There is no mention in the chapter that these conflicts involve a relationship between the parents, the child, and the health-care team, and most of the scenarios presented in the chapter consider the health-care professionals and parents only. In essence, then, the standard model of the physician-patient relationship has simply been shifted to the physician–parent relationship, with no consideration that the involvement of a child may require a new and different framework. In both these ways, by focusing on the adults involved and by focusing on the principles in question, the child is forgotten.

These moral systems leave no room for truly shared decision-making. While models for shared decision-making are increasingly viewed as the ideal in medicine, these models are developed with the adult patient in mind, and usually regarding a single medical issue. That is, the shared decision-making is predicated on a patient-physician dyad. These frameworks are insufficient for the complex and multifaceted needs of children at the end of life. Some look to the courts to decide between the desires of the parents and the desires of the medical care team, but the legal system is no better equipped to address the complex web of relationships in pediatric care. Nowhere does this become more obvious than in the entrenched conflicts that sometimes erupt between parents and health-care professionals, or within families themselves. These conflicts sometimes erupt into the public square, as with the recent cases of Charlie Gard or Archie Battersbee in the United Kingdom, where parents and health-care professionals ended up in court litigating different accounts of what was in the best interest of the children.

There is, moreover, little consideration about how including children in medical decision-making may require a whole new way of thinking about what it means to meaningfully participate—that there can be decisions that are neither mine nor yours, but properly *ours*. Nor is there consideration that what children reveal about humanity questions these frameworks of decision-making more broadly and fundamentally. It is important to question whether we need separate models for adults and children, or whether children reveal ways in which we are mistaken about our models writ large. Similarly, we need a framework that is not designed first and foremost, like many bioethical approaches, to deal with the "difficult questions," but one that can start from a place of cooperation and that considers not only specific actions, but the more nebulous types of decisions—those about meaning and about faith. This critique is not new, and several generations of theologians and theological ethicists have worked to re-situate medical decision-making, and decision-making more generally, within the broader scope of the human life. But so far, few have tackled the specific questions about the moral lives of children.

But whatever its faults, pediatric medicine is the only cultural force confronting and thinking about child death. In a society that actively ignores the voices of children, pediatric medicine has been thinking seriously about how to care for children with life-limiting illness. Myra Bluebond-Langner's groundbreaking work in a Baltimore leukemia ward in the 1970s showed that children can learn about their condition and respond to it in ways both meaningful and moral. Since then, physicians and researchers have been working to learn from children about how best to meet their needs. Pediatric medicine has transformed in the past century, from hospitals where parents would drop their children off and, hopefully, pick them up days or weeks later, to one in which some pediatric hospitals have adjoining rooms for parents so that they can share in the hospital life of their child. Pediatric medicine has excelled in bringing in so-called nonmedical personnel to contribute to the well-being of children. This is perhaps best exemplified in the role of child life specialists, whose job I once heard described as helping children to be children in the midst of their situation.

Similarly, it is often within pediatric ethics that critical questions about adult-centered decision-making models emerge. Much of the literature about children that I cite in this book comes from pediatrics. Many of the studies of children's ability to make decisions, to contribute meaningfully to their own care and care of others, and on the importance of speaking truth to children have emerged from *within* pediatric medicine. Children's hospitals have not only expanded research into childhood illness but have been instrumental in transforming the types of care children receive. I am deeply indebted to—and join my voice with—those clinicians, researchers, and ethicists who work to expose the ways in which the moral systems of medicine are adult-driven and fail to meet the needs of children, and who work to ameliorate the lives of dying children.

But while those specialists work pragmatically to adjust structures to better help children, I propose that what we need is a fundamental rethinking of the moral systems we have in place in medicine and in the wider culture. Pediatric medicine remains constrained by the systems of medicalization, by limited moral horizons, principlism, and the myopia of the physician-patient dyad. But it is not only pediatric medicine that needs to be confronted. Many of the challenges of pediatric care arise from the surrounding cultural ideas about children and childhood. When hospitals communicate with the public, the focus is on what can be achieved with medical technology. Take, for instance, the ad campaign "Versus" released by SickKids Toronto. The campaign's first advertisement video briefly shows a child flatlining, only for her to be quickly resuscitated to a triumphant soundtrack. Despite much criticism, for this and other reasons, the ad campaign continued to release videos and posters. Inspiring images of children overcoming illness sell. Compassionate care of the dying does not.

Many of the challenges of end-of-life care for and with children emerge because of the larger cultural stories of death avoidance and the underestimation of children's abilities that shape parental, familial, and patient attitudes. Physicians tend to only bring up palliative care if they perceive that a family is ready to accept that their child is going to die. A study published in 2021 compared the proportion of parents who talked about death with their dying children between 2001 and 2016.[13] These fifteen years were a time of significant change within pediatric medicine, from increasing advocacy for open communication at the end of life to open communication being the accepted norm in the field. Despite this, the study revealed no significant change in parental conduct. That is, despite that fact that we know children want to talk about death, and that open communication at the end of life helps children, parents, and families cope, there has been no meaningful change in behavior.

Decision-making at the end of life relies on larger cultural, philosophical accounts of what it means to be a person and what it means to make meaningful decisions. Thus, it needs to be *both within and without* the hospital that we reconsider what it means for a child to meaningfully participate in their medical care, and to engage in the process of dying. In a culture that avoids death, the medicalization of death allows society to relegate the dying child to a separate space—cut off, as it were, from the land of the living. These issues within pediatric care unite within a larger culture that diligently and effectively excludes children from the experience of, discussion about, or knowledge of death. For children to properly participate, we need to fundamentally reconsider their moral agency, to see them as able to live a good life and die a good death.

What is worse is that Christians, who are called to faith in God's love for children and in the resurrection of the dead, have conspired in the cultural silence around child death. This tragedy plays out in infrequent pastoral visits, depriving families of the prayers that have sustained dying Christians for centuries, of the presence of those who care about them, and of reminders of steadfast hope in the resurrection. Platitudes like "praying for a miracle" ignore the practical needs of children and their families. Christians too are complicit in behaviors like keeping children from visiting their sick friends in the hospital, as if somehow the knowledge of death makes it contagious. Children are not found in theological works on death, and in few pastoral manuals on death and dying. Many churches discourage children's attendance at funerals; some have even banned them. This conspiracy of silence means we are not teaching our children the stories of Christian hope in the face of death. It deprives a culture struggling with how to love and nurture children of the contributions that theological ideas about children can make.

Child death invites us to rethink simplified visions of childhood as merely a time of preparation for a "real" humanity. It forces us to confront the romantic notions of childhood innocence that persist in our thinking, and in our construction of "sacred" child spaces, which are cut off from the real world, as it were: spaces like nurseries, schools, family restaurants, and Sunday schools. Child death shows the insufficiency of these places. As amazing as pediatric hospitals are, they are not enough. They cannot provide the societal, cultural, and religious support so desperately needed by families and children with life-limiting illness. Child death invites us to recognize the ways in which children encounter tragedy, suffering, joy, challenges, and through all of this, make meaning with and for others, and for themselves.

This book takes up that invitation. We need to fundamentally rethink what it means for a child to live a good life and to die a good death. We need to situate children with life-limiting illness within a larger account of childhood that does not see it as simply a preparatory phase for "real life" and a time of innocence cut off from meaningful agency. We must think about children's agency within the hospital system as part of their broader morality. Children live complex lives in a complex world, one that includes serious illness and death. This failure to attend to children in the medical setting stems from a more general failure to recognize and understand the moral agency of children. It blinds parents, doctors, caregivers, and the wider public to what we can all learn from children, from their particular gifts for creating meaning, for affective response, and for asking questions that enrich our own lives. We grown-ups need to humble ourselves and listen.

∗∗

In light of these challenges, I propose to consider what it means for children to live a good life and die a good death. In this book, I argue that children are moral agents. Children act for themselves in the world, and they sometimes can and do act, especially with the help of others, *reasonably* for themselves in the world. Children's moral agency is grounded in their ability to make meaning, to act, to imitate, to use language creatively, to grasp a plurality of meanings, to reach judgments, to contribute to the meaning of others, and to shape their understanding. This agency is grounded in intersubjective subjectivity, and grounded in a particular story: where subjectivity, agency, and wholeness are found in the trinitarian God in whose image we are made.

This book considers children as moral agents beyond simple questions of decision-making capability, but as moral subjects who create meaning for themselves in the world, who have an account of good and evil, who learn to reason, and who contribute to the moral lives of others. That is, it considers moral agency beyond an account of decision-making to an account of the self. It considers the moral personhood of children in light of the stories we tell about children, the stories children tell (and we often fail to listen to), and the Christian story. These stories open alternate ways of knowing from "conventional" ways of knowing in bioethics, from a truncated account of action to a wholistic vision of the subject who acts.

In light of this, I argue that children can die a good death, and that they can and should have a voice in their end-of-life care. We ought to be honest with them and include them in decision-making. They can make real and meaningful choices around death. But to include children as moral agents requires changing how we understand moral agency and personhood, and challenging the liberal, individualistic, autonomous premises that underlie contemporary views of morality, especially when it comes to decision-making in medical contexts.

Thus, this book is also a sustained argument for children's participation in treatment decisions, especially in end-of-life decision-making. It is my contention that children can meaningfully contribute to so-called major decisions in medicine, such as DNR orders, cessation of life-prolonging care, amputations, and so on, as well as the more minor decisions, like location of treatment, funeral planning, symptom-management trade-offs, and what they want to have for lunch. Children are capable of participating in their medical care and decision-making. They can make decisions for themselves, and they can make decisions together with those around them. By considering these decisions in a larger framework of children's moral selfhood and agency, I hope to recognize the abilities of children while avoiding two errors: (1) that of seeing them as equal in capability to adults, and thus ignoring their development and the particular accommodations they need, and (2) ignoring the real capabilities they already have.

This book is aimed at two groups. The first and primary group consists of scholars and clinicians: theological ethicists, medical ethicists, and chaplains. It speaks to those who are interested in how we think about and pay attention to children in the medical setting. It addresses questions about how we express our experiences, understand our situations, arrive at reasonable conclusions, and make decisions. It challenges the narrow frameworks we have received about how capacity and agency are exercised in a medical setting, and the ways in which those frameworks exclude children from having input regarding their care. While theological ethicists often question autonomy, they focus on our responsibilities toward children and on moral issues surrounding fetuses and infants, and have little to say about the actual moral lives of children, or children's participation in moral reasoning.

This book's secondary and broader audience is those who are interested in moving beyond parenting blogs and pop psychology and want to think deeply about what it means to see children as full human beings, and the ways in which children, as full human beings, invite us to rethink our own ideas about what is central to the human person and the moral life. Looking upon the face of a child who will never grow up forces us to consider the meaning and value of childhood, not as the rehearsal for a future humanity, but as an end in itself.

This book is for anyone concerned with meeting children's particular needs without seeing them as non-persons or seeing them as identical to adults. This starts with a fundamental restructuring of what we think childhood is, and what we think of human life as a whole. It starts with eternal childhood, with seeing all human life in relationship as God's children. And so, this book is a project in *childism*, a conceptual reconstruction of our understanding of human nature in light of the dimensions of human meaning children reveal and the new horizons they open to us.

It should also be clear what this book is not. It is not a study of our obligations to confront starvation or a lack of access to medical care, nor is it about the plight of children in war-torn countries or those killed by natural disasters, though these too are important topics. I am not suggesting either that child death from starvation or widespread preventable disease around the world is a good thing, though I do believe that, even in those situations, children are moral agents who can make meaning in their deaths. This book is not a pastoral manual. I hope it encourages those who minister to children, including children with life-limiting illness, and challenges clerics and laypeople whose churches do not adequately pay attention to the experiences, voices, and needs of children. But it is not a how-to guide for talking to children or parents about death, and certainly any comments about the inability of parents or families or even physicians to confront death made in this book should not be used as a truncheon to chastise those perceived to be in the wrong.

✳✳✳

What, then, will I talk about in this book? I have begun by acknowledging that while pediatric hospitals are at the forefront of initiatives to include children in their own medical care, these efforts are hampered by ongoing cultural notions and moral structures that deny children's moral agency. In chapter 1, I ask: *How did we get here?* It has to do with both *who* we think are children and who we think *children are.* Our cultural impetus is to protect children from the evils of the "real" (i.e., public) world, not recognizing that children are already in the public world, that they are already affected by grief, sickness, inequality, and oppression. Ethical literature on children shares in the cultural confusion. Reflections on children tend toward one of two opposite assumptions: that there is and always has been a universalized notion of childhood, or that we are the first to recognize the true nature of children as children, and thus to value and love them. In fact, the history of childhood is long, complex, and heavily varied. There never has been, and still is not, a universalized account of childhood.

Where do we go from here? We must begin by confronting the confused and contradictory accounts of childhood latent in our culture. We must recognize that who is a child is a complex question. Childhood is socially constructed as well as biologically grounded. It is also theologically determined. Biblical witness challenges our existing ideas about childhood. Unlike stories involving adults, biblical stories about children are resoundingly positive. The treatment of orphans is the yardstick of Israel's faithfulness, and Jesus sets a child on his knee and holds her up as the model of discipleship—a theme that extends through the epistles as well. It is the little servant girl who directs Naaman where to seek healing for his leprosy, and a young boy who offers his lunch to Jesus, with which he will feed thousands.

Following Karl Rahner, I connect our identity as children of God to actual childhood: to grow in love and discipleship is to learn how to become a child of God. This journey begins in our actual childhood, where we are already in relationship with God, who, in the incarnate Son, became a child. To understand what this means, I suggest that we understand the *imago Dei* not as a particular capacity, like reason or language or creativity, but as intersubjectivity. It is from this intersubjective existence that all particular capacities arise. This is crucial for two reasons. First, because a lack of capacities has often been used to deny children a share in common humanity and participation in the moral world, and second, because approaches that focus on the humanity of children often cannot contend with growth and development, and so fail to highlight the importance of both nurturing and protecting children.

I propose that we understand the growth and development of children by seeing them as self-transcending subjects: they thirst for knowledge and for relationship with others. Children have particular gifts, what I call "goods of childhood"—curiosity, creativity, resilience, aptitude for learning, and flexibility, which are often lost or diminished with age. These gifts are shown, for example, in the ways in which children are held up as examples of discipleship in the New Testament. Children play a role in revealing what it means for all people to be children of God.

Acknowledging the shared humanity of children does not by itself pay sufficient attention to their moral lives. In chapter 2, *Can a Child Live the Good Life?* we must take the further step of recognizing that because children are *human* beings, they are therefore *moral* beings. We must reconceive of the fundamental aspects of human nature in light of children's shared nature, much in the same way that recognizing the inclusion of women, people of color, and people with disabilities has prompted a reconsideration of what it means to be human. This chapter presents an account of the moral agency of children, building on the understanding of children as intersubjective and self-transcending subjects introduced in the previous chapter.

Children should have some share in their decision-making not merely because they are the ones most affected, but rather because they are properly moral agents. Children make moral meaning, choose moral actions, and develop moral character. This does not mean that children are cognitively or morally identical to adults (an error made in recent efforts to increase children's participation by simply extending the right to decide to younger and younger children, an approach that still takes autonomy—the same autonomy that serves to dehumanize and exclude children—as the criterion of participation, and so fails to properly support or protect children). Children have particular gifts in the drive for knowledge of the good. It is our task as adults to recognize and nurture this ability. Children bring specific goods to the moral life. In their (often spontaneous) response to others, children call us to respond to their presence, actions, questions, and opinions, which can reveal to us the narrowness of our own moral deliberations.

In chapter 3, *Can a Child Die a Good Death?* I explore our understanding of death and dying as it relates to children. Nowhere is our desire to protect and nurture children so seemingly thwarted as in the case of a dying child. Few places so inhibit our ability to communicate love, to teach, to listen, to comfort, and to faithfully raise our children as the hospital room. Childhood seems antithetical to death. But recognizing the humanity of a dying child and properly caring for her necessitates confronting death, naming the sources of suffering, and confronting the moral and cultural barriers preventing us from recognizing that children can die a good death.

The notion of suffering may be universal, but the experience of suffering is never generic. In the case of children with life-limiting illnesses in Western, industrialized countries, there are particular sources of suffering that impact children who are dying. The witness of children can teach us how to confront and overcome these sources of their suffering. In so many creative ways, children make meaning in the dying process. Stories and fantasy are an especially potent way for children and adults to enter into conversations about death. Through nonsense (in the face of the mystery and unintelligibility of death), storytelling, presence, relationship, and dependence, children model the good death. Through these ways we can speak honestly with children about their pain, loneliness, and sorrow, allow them to freely express their suffering, and offer them comfort. Children have a range of feelings about themselves and their experiences of being ill. And these feelings are real, intentional responses to values that adults too often ignore. They often have specific desires for what happens at their funeral, or how their worldly goods will be distributed; children have a strong desire to care for those around them, to set all things in place. Listening to these desires, taking them seriously, and working alongside is part of caring for dying children.

The dying process is not inherently meaningless, and children are capable of finding meaning in death and dying. A good death is founded not on rational choice but on intersubjectivity, shared meaning-making, and presence; that is, on an encounter with those who are ill that does justice to who children are as human beings. Hope for a good death is found not in control and conscious choice, but in our relationships, in honest speech, in attending to the sources of suffering at the end of life, in the endless possibilities for meaning-making present in our lives and deaths, and in lament. As Christians, we know that our hope for both a good life and a good death is found in a life made complete through the intersubjectivity that is friendship with God.

In chapter 4, I ask *Does a Child Mean What She Says?* A significant impediment to properly addressing the needs of children in the medical system, and to including them in medical decision-making, is the lack of research into the experiences of children in the hospital. There is rampant cultural skepticism that children can accurately express their thoughts and feelings about themselves and death. The scope of their experiences is underestimated, and their capacity to accurately express these experiences is undervalued. However, when researchers have talked to children directly, they have discovered that, in fact, children as young as four or five had quite sophisticated understandings of death and dying. This realization, that children understand and grieve death, has led to slow but important changes in how we respond to and care for children in the face of death.

In order to listen to children and to conduct research into their experiences, we must see that children *can* meaningfully express their experiences. To see *how* this is the case, it is helpful to consider what we think experiences are, how they can be expressed, and how they are related to judgments of fact and judgments of value. Experience is not limited to certain bodily sensations or to emotions, but encompasses the whole person: bodily, emotionally, communally, aesthetically, and intellectually. The meaning of any idea or concept is not explicit and fixed, already out there in the world. It is not hidden in our experiences, waiting for language to display it accurately. The meaningfulness of a child's experience is generated in their attempts to symbolize it, both to themselves and to others. These attempts often take creative means—art or play—and are brought to fruition in the back-and-forth communication with others in which the experiences are further symbolized and interpreted. Imagination and art are ways in which children transform themselves and the world around them. They not only inherit meanings, but play with them, make new meanings out of old ones, and communicate these meanings to others. Because meaning can be shared and communicated in all these various ways, meaning-making allows for a collaboration, where the search for knowledge can be undertaken together.

Children are moral agents who can meaningfully express their experiences and make meaning even in the face of death, I argue in chapter 5, *Can a Child Choose?* In order to open up spaces for children to participate in medical decision-making, we must transform institutional structures that have traditionally excluded them.

Medical ethics is dominated by a principlist approach in which the threshold for participation relies on a capacity for rational consent, where what is rational is predicated on formal reason and literal language. Against a principlist view modeled on a binary relationship between patient and physician, I advocate for an approach that sees decision-making as a shared venture and part of the larger moral formation and broader moral agency of children. Including children in decision-making is not only appropriate for who they are as moral agents but will help mitigate issues of bias that accompany surrogate decision-making, and help parents and guardians make choices that properly take into account the experiences of the child patient.

Building on the work done in the preceding chapters, I claim that children are capable of meaningfully expressing what it is they want. The fact that children and adults share in the same moral world as each other means that this agency can be shared. Meaning is communicative; this communication can proceed asymmetrically, where a child communicates at the level of experience or desire, and an adult can interpret it in terms of a judgment and return that formulation to the child for confirmation. In this way, we can have meaningful shared decision-making. In exploring the moral agency that is grounded in the prior "we" of intersubjectivity, and involving communicative acts of meaning, we can move away from highly individualized accounts of decision-making in favor of a meaningful shared model.

Children want to be included in medical decision-making because they have something to say. But this does not mean they should be making these decisions *alone*. Seeing decision-making as a shared venture requires adults to critically reflect on their decisions, and to integrate insights and questions put forward by the child or children, and in this way it helps to mitigate the issue of bias. Importantly, since moral agency is formed in part by experience, the chance to be included in medical decision-making should not be sprung on children at the end of life but must be integrated from their first encounters with the medical system.

Addressing questions of decision-making at the end of life cannot avoid the question of child euthanasia. I address this in the epilogue. Enthusiasm for child euthanasia is gaining traction in many parts of the Western world, as traditional arguments against the intrinsic evil of the practice are no longer convincing to many. But existing arguments in favor of euthanasia are ultimately grounded in autonomy, that we construct our moral world for ourselves. But as I demonstrate repeatedly in this book, this same autonomy makes no room for children as moral agents. Thus, to reconfigure our account of the moral life to include children is also to undermine the foundation on which arguments for (and many against) euthanasia are predicated.

Given the research into all the ways in which we fail to engage with children, to properly attend to and treat their pain, to combat their isolation and fear, and especially given the ways in which children feel guilty about the burden of their illness on their parents, and their deep affective desire to comfort those they love, we ought first to name and confront these sources before declaring that the only option is termination of life. Dying children scare adults, and euthanasia should not be a quick fix for the genuine wish to ease their suffering. Instead, we must be willing to walk the dark road, to question our assumptions about the good life and the good death, to think deeply about who children are, what we owe them, and of what they are capable. We need to recognize them as moral agents, intersubjective and self-transcending subjects, and beloved children of God.

This book, then, will take many directions to consider more broadly how we envision the participation of children in the moral life. But at every stage this book is driven by the consideration of children who will never "grow up." It is an argument that sick and dying children should be both seen and heard, by their families, by their health-care providers, and by society. This investigation is grounded in the Christian story, informed by children who are dying and those who work with and study them, and imaginatively shaped by the stories that bring hope. It is an invitation to learn from Diamond and the many children like him. It is about learning to enter into the stories and fairy tales that enable us to imaginatively consider another way to live. It is about entering the story that enables all of us, from infancy to old age to, like Diamond, *befriend* death.

NOTES

1 George MacDonald, *At the Back of the North Wind*, (London: Alfred A. Knoff, 2001). The story is believed to be inspired by the death of MacDonald's son Maurice.
2 Cf. Marilyn Pemberton, "The Ultimate Rite of Passage: Death and Beyond in *The Golden Key* and *At the Back of the North Wind*," *North Wind* 27 (2008): 35.
3 Hugh Brody, "'The Deepest Silences': What Lies behind the Arctic's Indigenous Suicide Crisis," *The Guardian*. July 21, 2022. https://tinyurl.com/2dk92rvn.
4 Stanley Hauerwas, *God, Medicine, and Suffering* (Grand Rapids, MI: Eerdmans, 1990), 146.
5 Li Jalmsell et al., "On the Child's Own Initiative: Parents Communicate with Their Dying Child About Death," *Death Studies* 39 (2015): 115.
6 Allen Verhey, *The Christian Art of Dying: Learning from Jesus* (Grand Rapids, MI: Eerdmans, 2011), 173.
7 Gilbert Meilaender, *Bioethics: A Primer for Christians* (Grand Rapids, MI: Eerdmans, 2005), 102.
8 See Jo-Eileen Guylay, *The Dying Child* (Toronto: McGraw-Hill, 1978), Pamela S. Hinds et al., "Key Factors Affecting Dying Children and Their Families." *Journal of Palliative Medicine* 8 (2005): 70, Bluebond-Langner et al., "Preferred place of death for children and young people with life-limiting and life-threatening conditions: A systematic review of the literature and recommendations for future inquiry and policy," *Palliative Medicine* 27 (2013): 710.
9 Ulrika Kriecberg, "Why and Where do Children Die," *Acta Pædiatrica* 107 (2018): 1671.
10 Dietrich Niethammer, *Speaking Honestly with Sick And Dying Children & Adolescents: Unlocking the Silence*, trans. Victoria W. Hill (Baltimore: Johns Hopkins University Press, 2012), xiii.
11 Susan M. Turner and Gareth B. Matthews, "Introduction," in *The Philosopher's Child: Critical Essays in the Western Tradition*, eds. Turner and Matthews, (Rochester: University of Rochester Press, 1998), 1.
12 Bluebond-Langner et al., "Preferred place of death," 706
13 Ulrika Kriecsberg, "No impact of previous evidence advocating openness to talk to children about their imminent death," *Acta Paediatrica* (2021):1671–1672.

CHAPTER 1

Who Is a Child?

We are all children of God. What this means can only be understood in light of actual childhood. Actual childhood, in its turn, can only be understood in terms of our eternal relationship as God's children. Birth is a double beginning: We are born into the world as infants and children, and we are born as children of God. Children are born already in relationship with God and with others. We learn what it means to be a child of God in part by observing and recollecting childhood. Moreover, it is my contention that the goal of Christian discipleship is a second childhood that is understood in relation to our first childhood. This idea is the foundational conviction of this entire project. Because of this, "child" is *first and foremost a relational term* and only secondly an empirical one.

Critical examination of childhood as a relational term reveals that childhood is often defined in relation to what it is not—namely, adulthood. Attending to the oppositions set between childhood and adulthood is illuminating. Thus, what children are thought *not to be* is crucial in framing our understanding of childhood. Any examination of childhood must also consider the idealization of adult abilities and the goals of human life. But comparison and deconstruction only go so far. Primarily, to state that "child" is a relational term is to make a constructive argument: I propose that childhood must be understood in light of the human relationship to God and to others.

Answering the question "who is a child?" requires that we relate childhood to historical, biological, cultural, social, and theological understandings of children. Even though we must define childhood in light of our human relationship to God, it cannot be the case that theological considerations, divorced from context, determine who is a child. Our observations of children and their bodies, thoughts, and actions are what lead us to posit who they are theologically. Similarly, it is the cross-cultural and historical attention to children that challenges our poorly constructed theological ideals of childhood. Both societal changes and a shift in theological and philosophical thinking led thinkers like Jean-Jacques Rousseau to posit a stark divide between adults and children that we still hold to today.[1] Defining a child requires, then, a hermeneutical circle: these historical, cultural, and theological definitions are mutually informative. So while I begin this chapter by talking about historical and cultural understandings of children, it is not the case that I started with a biological and cultural definition of children and let these lead me to theological points.

Following Karl Rahner, I connect our identity as children of God to actual childhood: to grow in love and discipleship is to learn how to become a child of God. This journey begins in our actual childhoods, where we are already in relationship with God, in whose image we are made, and who, in the incarnate Son, became a child. To understand what this means, I suggest that we understand the *imago Dei* not as a particular capacity, like reason or language or creativity, but as intersubjectivity. It is from this intersubjective existence that all particular capacities arise. This is a crucial concept for two reasons. First, because a lack of capacities has often been used to deny children a share in common humanity and participation in the moral world, and second, because recent approaches in theology of children that focus on the humanity of children often cannot contend with their growth and development, and so fail to highlight the importance of both nurturing and protecting children in ever-changing ways.

I propose that we understand the growth and development of children by seeing them as self-transcending subjects, meaning they have an unrestricted desire for knowledge, truth, and goodness, and for relationship with others. Children have particular gifts, what I call "goods of childhood": curiosity, creativity, resilience, aptitude for learning, and flexibility, which are often lost or diminished with age. These gifts are shown, for example, in the ways in which children are held up as examples of discipleship in the New Testament. Actual children play a role in revealing what it means for all people to be children of God.

This porous interplay between our first childhood and what I am calling our second or enduring childhood that characterizes Christian discipleship is at odds in a legal and political culture that is moving toward a more rigid and universalizing definition of "child" as all those under the age of 18. This definition ignores the significant different cultural and philosophical conceptions of childhood. I suggest that attention to actual, lived childhood reveals it to be not rigid and self-contained, but intrinsically porous and multivalent. Childhood spills into all areas of life, both a beginning and a goal of human maturity. So to understand the theological points I make in this chapter, it is helpful first to look at cultural and biological definitions of "child," to see how the rigid boundaries of childhood, seemingly so objective and empirical, are formed through the interplay of biological characteristics and cultural meaning.

This claim, that child is a relational term, does not discount the obvious biological differences between children and adults, from those to which we ascribe little significance—like the number of bones or surface-to-body-weight ratio—to those, like brain plasticity and size, to which we ascribe incredible importance. But these differences do not on their own provide a particular view of childhood. Instead, historical and cross-cultural childhood studies demonstrate the ways in which "biological immaturity is assigned social meanings dependent on the cultural setting."[2] These social meanings can in turn influence what is seen as biologically determined behavior. Anthropologist Heather Montgomery describes how the turbulence of toddlerhood or adolescence, generally ascribed in Western countries to the rapid biological (and thus universal) changes of those periods, is not universal. In some cultures, neither period of life is described or experienced by children and their families as any different than the gradual growth of young life.[3]

In the next section of this chapter, I will talk about the social meanings we have ascribed to biological immaturity in Western Europe and North America, especially, but not limited to, anglophone regions. This study is necessarily selective, focusing on those social meanings that are most pertinent to the inclusion of children in meaningful decision-making surrounding their deaths. It is especially pertinent because it is largely a Western European and North American view of children that is represented in the universalizing definition of children as all those under the age of 18, and as having their own separate rights and responsibilities. This is exemplified in the 1989 United Nations Convention on the Rights of the Child, where these definitions are found and which, incidentally, involved no children in the eleven-year process of being drafted.[4]

In today's confused cultural conversation about children, one thing is clear: childhood as a cultural entity is primarily defined in opposition to adulthood. Nostalgia plays a role here, as certain aspects of childhood are given a romanticized and outsized role. Adulthood is a time of moral and economic responsibility; childhood is thus a time of innocence and consumption. Adulthood is active and participatory, childhood is sheltered and protected. Irrational versus rational, sexually ignorant versus sexually active, home versus public sphere: in all of these ways, childhood is conceived as being *not adulthood*. One of the main issues with this universalizing childhood is that it sets the ideal of humanity—and thus the account of moral agency, political participation, cognition, and even subjectivity—according to the idealized and largely imagined adult, as if adulthood is a static period of life. This perspective is replicated in developmental psychology, where these assumptions underpin the establishment of norms and measurement of children's abilities.[5]

Notions of innocence and irresponsibility bely the reality that children already can and *do* act for themselves in the world. Take, for instance, the statement that play is the work of children. What, then, of the play of adults? Or the work of children? This is predicated on a narrow definition of each that then requires analogical links to understand. There is the thing that adults do: that is work. And it is, in contrast, anti-child for children to work. This has long been the position of activists campaigning against child labor. Similarly, the view that play is essentially childish allows work, the defining adult characteristic, to dominate adult life. This is bad for a number of reasons and redefines leisure time as the pursuit of other "worthwhile" things. It is also a universalizing view, ignoring that childhood's relation to play is culturally specific. It also tends toward a devaluation of play as simply an imitation of or preparation for adult work. In many cultures, like those of the Inuit, for example, play functions importantly in adult life and relationships. And studies of children's play suggest it is a way to transform and transcend social realities, including conflict and tragedy.[6]

This oppositional relationship is reflected in the cultural persistence of the charge that previous cultures saw children as small adults.[7] Although this concept has been debunked by historians, I believe this idea endures because those cultures ascribed to children's behaviors and responsibilities that which we think anathema to childhood: work, participation in public life and religious ritual, sexual maturity of adolescents, and so on. If childhood is defined as ignorant and innocent, and characterized by relegation to the sanctified space of the home and school, and if this understanding of childhood is universal, then it must be that other times and places had no account of childhood.

These dominant universalizing accounts of children's selfhood and moral agency define childhood in relation to *not adulthood* because they do not begin with the study of the beginning of agency in a child's life. Psychologists find that infants as young as three months can morally differentiate.[8] Instead, childhood is measured on a romanticized deficiency model, as lacking a vision of moral agency that considers only a small population of adults as the baseline. Educational policies, focused on what a child ought to become, are also models of dependency, reifying the notions of childhood helplessness and ignorance. They state that the goal of childhood is to *become* good adults who can then act in the world. Except in a few educational circles, there is little sense that children can help confront the challenges of this life in cooperation with adults. There is little sense that children can contribute, not as romantic heroes wiser than those around them, but as actual humans who have something to teach us even as they learn. But as I will talk about at the end of this chapter, the particular gifts of children serve to complement adult abilities.

None of this is to say that there are not differences between infants, children, adolescents, young adults, those of middle age, and the elderly. In fact, those differences are key if we are to talk about goods of childhood, or of any stage of life. These differences also mean that children are in need of protection and accommodations in order to be treated with equality in the world. But our cultural impetus to protect children from the evils of the "real" (i.e., public) world means that we often fail to recognize that children are already in the public world, that they are already affected by grief, sickness, inequality, and oppression. Protection often amounts simply to exclusion. Increasing aversions to the risk of certain types of harms (all accidents can be prevented!) often means protection trumps participation. For example, in my home country of Canada, children are excluded from some Parliament buildings because there are no railings or other safety equipment. This rule does not consider the harms that come from the exclusion of children from having any influence, through their presence and words, in the laws and policies that govern their lives.

To confront the ways in which we define childhood in opposition to adulthood is crucial to understand what it means for children to model a proper relationship to God. In addition, if what it means to be a child of God is in part shaped by our observation and recollection of actual childhood, it is important to understand the cultural forces that bias this observation. By challenging the stark divide between children and adults, we can see the ways in which children are already in the world and affected by its evils. By attending to what children have to teach us, we can fruitfully explore ways in which humans of all ages can work together to confront these realities. The theological belief that childhood is a double beginning requires that we begin this exploration of humanity, as it were, at the beginning: to consider humanity as it begins in relationship to others and to God.

✳✳✳

Let us begin by asking ourselves: Who is a child? When we do this, it becomes instantly apparent how easy and difficult it is to answer this question. In one sense, we all know who is a child. Look around you! We see children in our homes, in schoolyards, in the grocery store. To ask, "Who is a child?" is to ask the obvious.

But unpacking the definition of child and childhood proves difficult. In this section, I will look to actual childhood, as it is conceptualized, and how it is lived and experienced. It is important to confront the confused and contradictory accounts of childhood latent in our culture, stemming from the legacy of Victorian bourgeois visions to post-industrial romantic idealization of childhood innocence to educational theories of taming or shaping children to capitalist systems which place the value of children in the production or consumption of goods. We must recognize that "Who is a child?" is a complex question. As Erica Burman puts it so perfectly, children are "a site of investment for all kinds of hopes, fears, and longings."[9]

Childhood is socially constructed as well as biologically grounded. In our culture, we have a tendency to define childhood primarily by age groups, letting certain so-called empirical and biological categories determine what it means to be a child. But these definitions depend on a compartmentalization of human experience into two fundamentally different things—childhood and adulthood—that have little to do with each other, while at the same time instrumentalizing childhood according to the goals of a capitalist, democratic citizenry. It is hard to escape our cultural ways of thinking, so here I will bring up examples from other times and other places for two reasons: (1) to help us see how our cultural notion of childhood is more diverse than we think, and (2) to investigate some of the latent ideas in contemporary Western society about children.

The definition of a child that dominates child policy publications, government websites, and NGO statements of purpose, is the definition found in the United Nation's 1989 Convention on the Rights of the Child (UNCRC): a child is anyone under the age of 18. The UNCRC does not mention adolescence. This definition functionally separates humanity into two groups: children, who fall under the definition, policies, and protections of childhood, and adults, the model of self-actualized citizenship. This view, rooted in particular cultures and associated with particular philosophical beliefs, has been reinforced in medicine and developmental psychology, such that this arbitrary division has taken on the pall of objective and empirical fact.

This simple definition, that a child is anyone under 18, does not itself explicitly name the cultural meanings that shape and accompany the definition. It is largely the field of childhood studies, by observing children across cultures and through history, as well as studying the poor and nonconforming others in our societies, that has named the elements of this so-called universalized account of childhood: *innocence, fragility and thus protection, consumption and thus economic burden, irresponsibility, submission, and sexual ignorance.*

This "universal" account of childhood has largely undervalued the abilities of children and stripped them of their place in larger society, sequestered them within individual private homes, and pathologized them if they end up in circumstances that deviate from this norm (as in the case of children who work or who have sex). Against the universalizing account of childhood that dominates the UNCRC and Western policy-making more generally, developmental psychology, and the Western imagination, it is the dominant view in childhood studies that childhood is constructed in the interplay of biological and cultural realities or, as Montgomery puts it, "biological immaturity is assigned social meanings dependent on the cultural settings."[10]

That there are different ways of thinking about children does not mean they are equally correct. In fact, the issue with the universalizing account of childhood is that it ignores or downplays many elements of childhood in favor of a few. Ideally, we would shape our ideas of childhood in part by observing actual children, by encountering them as others with different bodies and dynamic physiology, who rapidly grow and develop in conversation with our cultural and religious values and our accounts of humanity more generally. But in reality, our observations of childhood are often determined by our accounts of humanity writ large, and our culture's place for children. That is, we only see what we intend to see.

It cannot be the project of this book to give a review of childhood studies and the history of childhood, but this inter- and trans-disciplinary work is vast and enlightening, and I must content myself with a brief and simplified account, focusing on the elements most pertinent to the topic of this book. This means I will focus on the ideas about childhood that lead to the failure to see children as affected by the harms of exclusion, and the inability to acknowledge their agency and contributions. Historical and cross-cultural approaches show us it is simply not true that childhood has only recently existed. Both childhood studies and theological reflection call into question elements of this universalized, limited, and sequestered childhood. In order to understand the vision of children laid out in the later sections of this chapter, it is important to talk about the cultural ambivalence toward children, and especially to confront the notions of childhood innocence and vulnerability that serve to undervalue and sequester them.

It is hard to overestimate the impact of the Enlightenment and the Victorian images of childhood as a time of innocence, fragility, consumption, irresponsibility, play, submission, and sexual ignorance. The eighteenth and nineteenth centuries set in motion changes in the view of children that still impact Western culture today, especially in the anglophone world. Against the backdrop of the Industrial Revolution and the Enlightenment, and in response to the rampant child labor in factories, burgeoning ideas about workers' rights and new definitions of the person went hand in hand with a changing understanding of the child. These changes were philosophical, theological, and social. In the span of a century or two, children were expelled from the "adult business of modernity," relegated and sequestered to the private sphere of the home and schools.[11] Importantly, historians trace loss in the value of children in the "real world," such that children are assets (or burdens) to individual parents rather than contributing members of society writ large. Those parents, meanwhile, should make sure that they are financially prepared to take on the economic and emotional burden of child-rearing, since it is *their* business. It is only in such a cultural logic, for example, that the accusation of selfishness aimed at people who desire to have children or, shockingly, more than one or two, can make sense.

Conversely, the emotional value of children within the individual family came to take primacy of place, and significant focus was given to adequate emotional nurture, especially prizing sacrificial models of unconditional mother love. Care for children was no longer seen as a broad cultural task, but one of individual families. This model of proper love for children has significantly impacted Western views of poor and of so-called primitive cultures and provided the basis for arguing that they do not sufficiently love their children. Similarly, it allowed for the significant (ongoing) exploitation of poor children and the regulation of parents, especially mothers, according to policy shaped by an overestimation of parental agency and limited exploration of the impact of larger social structures on the lives of children.[12]

It is to Jean-Jacques Rousseau that we owe the first articulation of childhood as a sphere of life cut off from that of adults, sequestered away, pure, natural, and untainted.[13] Both he and his contemporaries saw children as "quasi-divine ... [the] embodiment of natural innocence."[14] The association of childhood with purity and innocence was not entirely new; ancient Athenians and medieval Christians, among others, both saw in children an element of purity, though this was held in tension with their undeveloped, wild, and sinful nature.[15] But in the Enlightenment period, it became the norm that children, now viewed as qualitatively other, should be sequestered away from society, protected from the adult world. Childhood was endowed with its own sets of values and goals. This was true of some developmental accounts of childhood too. This change was driven, at least in part, by changes in the wider culture. With the rise of urbanization and industrialization, children were not only working in households and on farms, but increasingly under exploitative conditions in factories and mines. As the wider society changed, so did children's participation in it, and the nurture and education they had previously received in the home became rare. It is no wonder, then, that there was a move made to protect them, to sequester them away, and to prioritize education.

Emerging educational frameworks in the eighteenth and nineteenth centuries were modeled on the existing and developing ideas about epistemology and the goals of education. In this way, views of childhood were tied to emerging beliefs about evolution. Evolution, for many thinkers of the period, became an explanatory framework not only for nonhuman life-forms, but could be replicated in human cultures and in the life of the individual. This thought was explicitly ageist and racist: "The highest stage of evolution was the European adult male while the savage and the child were at the bottom of the hierarchy."[16] This framework was repeated in terms of rationality and epistemology; that is, what types of knowledge were acceptable, verifiable, true—the positivism that shaped Enlightenment intellectual pursuits—and what types of knowledge did not pass muster—the mythical, story, nonempirical. Thus there emerged a twin dejection and romanticization of "primitive" knowledge, whether in the individual child or in childish cultures.

These evolutionary beliefs were also reflected in public health initiatives. The social hygiene movement is noteworthy for its impact on improved care for children, and especially in the decrease in child mortality seen in the Victorian period. But it was tied up with the cultural aspirations of developed nations.[17] If children were the future of these civilized nations, children with deformities or other disabilities were not viewed as representative of that cultural superiority. Increased cultural treasuring of children did not often extend to mentally handicapped or disfigured children and there is a long, terrible, and only recently abandoned (for the most part) history in medicine of experimenting on unwanted children and those with physical or cognitive disabilities.[18] Similarly, Burman and Montgomery both see the social hygiene movement as a significant origin for the pathologization of poor parents, especially mothers, and the rising trust in expert advice over familial experience when it comes to correct forms of child-rearing. To previous generations, the idea that there was one way to raise a child, and that a wholly unconnected person would know how to raise a child better than one's own parents and grandparents, would be largely unthinkable.

This is in no way to suggest that these changes were wholly bad. As always, there is a push and pull between the benefits and downsides. The social changes that arose in the Enlightenment, which included improving care of foundlings, educating mothers on care for infants, improving economic and social conditions, and providing women with means to reduce the number of children they bore, led to a sharp decline in infant and child mortality between the early eighteenth century and the early nineteenth century.[19] Similarly, curbing exploitative child labor and expanding publicly funded education improved the lives of countless children. For all the downsides of the romanticization of childhood, the Enlightenment approach was helpful insofar as it drew attention to who children are as children.

The changes of this time period also meant that children's lives became increasingly defined by bureaucratization, something that continues today. Children are more and more defined by the year in which they were born, through division under specific government policies and, more prominently, by education. Children today are thought of in relation to their age and their grade, and relationships between children are defined by these rigid categories of "cohort." With the decline of intergenerational meeting spaces and, in many places, concern about letting children explore on their own together without adult supervision, these categories become more rigid, with significant impact on children's growth and development. As this happens, we become more and more dedicated to standards that dictate what "normal" children of a certain age can achieve. It is a marker of the way bureaucratization and the resulting numerical categories have taken preeminence that the United Nations definition of a child mentions only a number as the definitional element, and not even particular physical elements, nor rational capabilities, nor cultural or religious factors.

It was this penchant for statistics and bureaucratization, as well as changing views of childhood, that led to the medical specialization of pediatrics. In other words, the physiological differences between children and adults took on new cultural meaning. For a variety of reasons, medical practitioners came to realize that adult-centered care did not apply easily to children and began to develop hospitals and care that suited the differences between children and adults—where adolescents fit into this scheme has always presented a problem. This bureaucratization united developmental psychology with pediatrics and education: In the clinic and school, children could be weighed, measured, and compared to emerging norms in various categories, which, in turn, furthered the idea that these measurements contain significant meaning about childhood. Thus, the pediatric clinic became the arbiter of normal childhood development, and developmental milestones structured the way in which parents observe their children.

This focus on bureaucratically defined ages combined with development goals predicated on the independent male adult meant that developmental studies of children's abilities in psychology and even sociology were undertaken according to the models of idealized moral agency and rational capability. Children's abilities were measured according to how well they measured up to this goal. There is a focus on what a child can achieve alone, rather than collaboratively, and in comparison to an idealized adult. Sociology and psychology have long evaluated child development through a "polarization between childhood and adulthood" where the child was a "substantial other."[20] One scholar calls this "generationing," akin to "gendering," where certain common attributes of a given age take on an essentialized view of what every child of that age can or cannot do.

Medicine and psychology shape much of the cultural imagination around childhood today. But as Burman depicts in her book on developmental psychology, cultural, philosophical, and political ideas about children shape the ideas psychologists bring to their work, and the types of questions they ask. These influential disciplines are still impacted by the relegation of children to the private realm, and so consider the child primarily in the individual context of the nuclear family, and rarely investigate any link between a child and the wider social and political context. It is significant, then, that most developmental psychology studies come from one country.[21] These psychological conceptions of childhood are powerful and exert a lingering hold on the culture, even if the field is now taking on a relational approach and considering the critiques of childhood studies. This is because we internalize and institutionalize these norms and pass them on to our children. They shape parental, educational, and cultural action.

The perspectives of the eighteenth and nineteenth centuries also shape contemporary theological reflection on children through the dominance of an unhelpful trifold typology found in contemporary theology of children. This typology divides theological views of childhood into three categories: top-down or original sin, bottom-up or natural good, and developmental or *tabula rasa*.[22] This typology divides contemporary and historical theological views of childhood into three categories and reads into the past particular and oversimplified views of Kant, Rousseau, and Locke. Because of its universalizing tendencies, this typology skews evaluation of historical theological and biblical texts. For example, Jesus and Schleiermacher get lumped together in opposition to Paul and Calvin. These are not actually three universal ways of seeing children, but belong to a certain cultural moment, albeit one with enduring power. It is also why this typology fails when applied to pre-Enlightenment thinkers, whose notions of childhood are qualitatively different.

There is no question that we live in the shadows of the significant changes to the notion of childhood in the modern period. Especially, we live in the legacy of Rousseau, whose romantic vision of childhood caught the cultural imagination. Children have lost visibility and value in the public sphere. Children are, especially in a moral sense, romanticized. Pushbacks against corporal punishment, and against harsh methods of upbringing and their roots in the theological notion of original sin, have created an atmosphere in which children are viewed as amoral, or innocent.[23] We live in the legacy of these ideals; the agency of children today is disregarded, and children are pushed to the margins of society.

If all of this sounds like an Enlightenment fall paradigm, it is not. In the first place, I am not advocating a paradisical view of childhood in the centuries preceding this period. The focus on rationality as the marker of humanity, isolated and elevated in the Enlightenment, has its roots in theological and philosophical thinking through at least two millennia prior. And while children did have broader support through their communities and more rights and responsibilities as adolescents, there were also many deaths of mothers too young to safely bear children and, especially in cities, a precarity among poor and disabled children that far exceeds today and was a key reason for the establishment of bureaucratized child services. And even where children enjoyed more broad communal support, they were still vulnerable to forces outside their communities, like famine and war. There is no going back to a "glorious age."

Similarly, some of the factors I identify as stemming from the Enlightenment do not result in significant changes during that time but are the beginning of practices common in the twentieth and twenty-first centuries. Chief among these is the use of child policies in global diplomacy. For example, monetary aid is often contingent on foreign countries adopting particular policies about children that ignore local cultural meaning. Teenage refugees who are able to travel miles must be received into Western countries under child laws, and thus must exchange their rights and responsibilities in order to receive protection. Other changes are mitigated. While Western children are still sequestered, they do have increased rights of participation in public life, even if this is predicated on a divide between proto- and actual citizenship.

In twenty-first-century North America, our view of children is controlled in new ways by the logic of market utility: children are products, reflections of the success of their parents.[24] Not only are children used and manipulated to serve the ends of their parents, but this view encourages other children to be viewed primarily as competitors, not as companions or as others in whom we have a vested interest. Bonnie Miller-McLemore and Joyce Ann Mercer both point out that as well as being treated as products, children are increasingly targeted as prime consumers.[25] But children as products and children as consumers do not exhaust the logic of market utility. In the logic of market utility, children must primarily be burdens—those who not only fail to contribute to the market but who reduce the productivity of their parents and other adult caregivers. It is in this kind of environment that philosopher Harry Adams can see a sick child as reducing the autonomy of her parents.[26]

The three areas where children are most commonly used and commodified are war, sex, and work—with child soldiers, child prostitution, and child labor—which, while societally condemned in the Western world, remain a common phenomenon worldwide.[27] Thus, in contemporary society, our view of children is a confused combination of these views: the child as innocent, amoral, and sequestered, but also as consumer and competitor. Children are economically burdensome but have high emotional value in the eyes of parents. It also means that the focus of parenting is intensive nurturing of abilities, which in turn is given a heightened importance in the competitive capitalistic world. These abilities, in turn, are measured according to capitalist ideals: conformity is conflated with maturity.[28]

Childhood studies, an academic field made up of scholars from a variety of disciplines, focuses on the lived experiences of children across cultures, times, and places. This research has demonstrated that children display different emotional expression, interpersonal abilities, skills, capabilities, and contributions to family and social life. They view their own behavior and responsibilities in various ways. Held up to historical and cross-cultural scrutiny, the images of childhood as a time of innocence, fragility, consumption, irresponsibility, play, submission, and sexual ignorance do not hold muster. In fact, this view has only ever represented a small percentage of children both in the Victorian period and today. Those children who fit the protected, sequestered life, largely due to economic privilege, were innocent and wise; those who did not were amoral, animal-like, and in need of constraint.

This romanticizing and pathologizing continues today, and the concept of child is still used rhetorically to indicate moral blamelessness. This is striking in its gendered, racial, and classist elements. If childhood is relational to what it is not, then boys must throw away the qualities of childhood to become men. So boys must "take on the attributes of responsibility, dominance, and virility."[29] Because of this, older boys, especially teenage boys, are viewed with deep moral suspicion. Girls do not face the same expectations, and so girlhood tends to extend much further. For example, there is a habit in public and moral discourse to speak of teenage girls as children.

One example is the use of the term "child bride," which conjures up images of prepubescent girls being wed against their will. But often the term is used to describe teenagers who are of the age of consent. Similarly, our society tends to view teenage mothers as transgressive. This is despite the fact that most children in the world are born to women below the age of 20. I don't mean to imply that age boundaries are rigid between cultures (i.e., one can be a teen in one place and an adult in the other), but issues around capabilities should be in the least relative. In contrast, teenage boys are no longer spoken of as children. While newspapers and government policies happily talk about 17-year-old girls as child brides, no one talks about a 17-year-old male shooter as a child. Interestingly, this gender dynamic stands opposite to many historical views, in which girls transitioned to womanhood at puberty, ready for their lives as wives and mothers. Boys, on the other hand, who matured (on average) physically later and who were to have an education did not become men, marked by marriage and a profession, until significantly later.

Notably, in most cultures across history and even in many parts of the world today, genital development and puberty play a key role in the transition from childhood to adolescence (or even adulthood). In contemporary Western culture, the stark divide between child and adult has led to a functional loss of an adolescence that differs significantly from childhood in terms of home life or societal rights and responsibilities. There is an important difference between a child and an adolescent having sex, or working, or making legally binding decisions—though acknowledging this difference does not mean approving these actions.

While puberty should not be a sole arbiter of transition from childhood, adolescents should have increased decision-making rights and responsibilities that correspond with their growth and development. Some institutions are beginning to recognize this fact; although policy makers adopt the United Nations definition of child as anyone under the age of 18, bodies within the organization, like the World Health Organization, push for adolescence as a separate category, and for the inclusion of adolescents under labor organizations.[30] However, the main place this category is used is in court cases. In many places, children and youths are referred to collectively as children under pornography and immigration laws, but separately under criminal justice laws.[31] The stage of adolescence should be recognized in legal frameworks for children's participation, and not just for punishment.

So we can see that our current way of thinking about two distinct stages of life—childhood and adulthood—is an outlier, and the universalizing simplified definition of child as anyone under 18 ignores vast differences between children of different ages, and between cultural categories. Julie Faith Parker finds almost thirty words used to describe children and youth in the Hebrew Bible.[32] The Ancient Greeks divided life into "two, three, four, five, six, seven, and even ten stages, based on numerology or astrology, the number of seasons or of fingers on each hand," and the terms used were elastic.[33] What is notable about these schemes is that they also divide adulthood into multiple stages, rather than seeing it as a static entity. If childhood is defined in part by what it is not, then a plethora of life stages to compare it with softens the differences and enhances the sense of continuity. Instead of irrational, irresponsible child versus rational, responsible adult, we have childhood as different in small ways from youth, from early adulthood, from middle age, from the twilight of middle age, from elderly, from old, from ancient.

I want to encourage this use of varied terminology of infant, baby, toddler, child, tween, teen, adolescent, young adult, and so on to discuss those who fall under the broad umbrella of child, as it is commonly conceived. I believe that there is no reason to hold to a strong divide at age eighteen, or any age, between children and adults. Certainly, while this stark divide dominates legal and policy documents, the age of transition is not consistent in our culture: the age of drinking, sexual consent, and age at which one can vote or give legal consent are not the same in most jurisdictions. Instead of seeing this as a bad thing, I think that it is entirely appropriate that these stages are reached at different ages in different contexts, that different facets of adulthood are achieved at different times, and that what we consider facets of adulthood may more properly be facets of adolescence or childhood as well. I hold that there are ways in which children are qualitatively different than adults, but only in a soft sense; there is no clean divide between child and adult, and certainly the two are not opposed in the many ways—innocence versus responsibility, development versus stasis, passivity versus agency—that underpin so much thinking about children today.

In this book, I focus on those who more narrowly fit the term *children*: those roughly under the age of twelve, mainly between the ages of three and twelve. I am thinking especially of those who have been weaned, who use language, but who have not yet reached or are only just reaching puberty. In more cultural terms, I'm referring—roughly—to those who attend preschool and elementary school. I am using the word "roughly" for two reasons. First, as in any categorization, the margins are difficult to define. Language acquisition, walking, and puberty happen at different times from child to child and, statistically speaking, between the sexes, but they mark important points of transition. Second, the word "roughly" denotes that I do not intend to create a stark divide between categories. Infancy, childhood, and adolescence are not discrete units or stages with no overlap or influence on each other, but names to help demarcate different stages of human development. The word "roughly" is meant as a reminder that the category of childhood, while existing and capable of being given a definition, is not absolute.

The lives of children are varied and multifaceted. They exist in many cultural matrices. There is no universal definition of child. But it is certainly not true, when attending to the lives of actual children, that childhood is a time of irresponsibility, innocence, fragility, and ignorance. A child is a relational and social being, who exists in a matrix of relationships that are both private and public (insofar as that distinction exists). Children develop in relation to their biology, their cultural context, and their familial setting. And, as I will discuss in the following section, childhood is porous and part of our whole life, not in a single deterministic way, but properly enduring. Children have significant abilities, goods of childhood, that have something to teach us about what it means for all people to be children of God.

***

If childhood is a double beginning, then it must be understood in light of both actual childhood and eternal childhood in God. In the first section of this chapter, I wrote about how our culture thinks of actual childhood, including the ways in which we unhelpfully divide adulthood and childhood into two qualitatively different stages that are understood in opposition to each other. Similarly, I questioned the notion of childhood as a time of irresponsibility and innocence. These criticisms are crucial for understanding what it means to be a child of God. If we take a romantic model of sequestered innocence, we fail to understand this goal of divine childhood, and what children have to teach us about what it means to be a human being created by God. If we do not recognize that children already share in the same world, and that they can (and do!) act for themselves, we miss that we can learn from them a certain stance toward the world and God. Attending to how human life begins tells us something about what it means to be children. But childhood does not speak for itself, as if its meaning existed already out there, uncontested, waiting only to be uncovered. What it means to be a child can only be understood in the context of what it means to be created in the image of God, what it means for God to be Father, and what it means to be united to his eternal Son in relationship with the Holy Spirit.

Instead of seeing childhood as the opposite of the adult ideal, childhood should be understood in the context of the ideal of Godly childhood. This lens lets us attend to the particular elements of actual childhood without descending into denigration or romanticization, or simply finding a *via media* in developmental accounts. Thus, I did not simply turn to childhood studies to determine who a child is. Instead, my critique and questions of common Western notions of childhood are framed by my theological viewpoint. Indeed, the central theological claim that I am making is not found in childhood studies.

My claim is this: childhood is also the *goal* of human life. It is only when we strip away the romanticized innocence of childhood that we can see that "childhood faith is 'already and inevitably' conditioned by the 'guilt, death, suffering, and bitterness' of human life."[34] And it is only when we understand childhood as the goal of human life that we can appreciate the strengths children bring to our lives, especially in collaboration with each other, and with guidance from others.

Story provides an imaginative entryway into this concept. George MacDonald's fairy tale *The Golden Key* has deeply shaped my own understanding of childhood as a double beginning, and as the goal of life. In the story, a little girl, Tangle, and a boy, Mossy, embark on a journey together to find the door that can be opened by the titular key.[35] Mossy, though a child, accepts the responsibility of this quest when he comes upon the key by chance while searching for the place where the rainbow ends. The young-looking woman who initially sends Tangle and Mossy on their quest is, in fact, thousands of years old. As they embark on their search for the door, they meet the Old Man of the Sea, the Old Man of the Earth, and the Old Man of the Fire—the oldest of them all. In the fiery center of the Earth, they find that this oldest of all men is a baby. Through the story, though it seems to Tangle and Mossy that it takes only a few days, Tangle becomes an old woman, gray and wrinkled. Yet at the end of the story, after being separated from each other, Mossy and Tangle reunite, and Mossy finds her looking young, much like the wise woman who took them in at the start. The child and the childlike are intertwined in this story, and through reading it we come to understand that it is the same in the world around us. Tangle and Mossy age as we ought to: First they are children, then adults, and then they revert to youth, but a youth that is wise.

Biblical stories also help to shape our imagination. From the beginning, the biblical narrative includes children in what it means to be made in the image of God. In the story of Seth, Adam and Eve's son, the repetition of image and likeness language from the creation story demonstrates that this continues even after the fall and expulsion from Eden. Throughout the Bible, children are integrally part of God's work in the world. The Abrahamic promise is predicated on the gifting of children. God's ability to overcome the barrenness of Sarah, Rebekah, and Rachel all reinforce this promise.[36] These miraculous conceptions are a reminder that children are a gift from God and not simply a product of human action. In turn, children are to be valued and brought up in knowledge of the covenant.[37]

The conviction, stemming from scriptural narratives, that children share fully in the *imago Dei* is a central hallmark of the theology of children. Children are not animals, not proto-humans, but already fully human. Image-of-God language is a central way that theologians and biblical scholars—and Christians more generally—speak of the dignity and value of all children. Central to this belief is Jesus's call to welcome children: "Whoever welcomes one of these little children in my name welcomes me; and whoever welcomes me does not welcome me but the one who sent me." The message of Jesus is that children have primacy of place in the kingdom of God.

But how we define what it means to be created in the image of God has a significant impact on how we view humanity, and how we envision children's (full) participation in that image.[38] Recognizing children as equal sharers in the *imago Dei* requires a reevaluation of how we understand the image of God. A whole range of definitions has been offered for the *imago Dei*, including cognitive and spiritual endowments like rationality and intelligence, an immortal soul, the ability to make moral decisions, language, love, response to beauty, relationship to God.[39] Recent works in theology of children have critiqued theology for its focus on rationality as the marker of the *imago Dei*, seeing as it excludes children (among others) from full participation in the image. Against this, childist theologians have chosen capacities that better include children: creativity and vulnerability.[40]

But predicating the image of God on any particular capacity risks excluding people from full participation in the image, and this remains true even for reimagined capacities. Like rationality, creativity has varied definitions and while children clearly excel in the immediate and spontaneous experience of seeing something in a different way, it is not clear that they demonstrate the same ability for sustained and ordered creativity, like that required to write Dante's *Divine Comedy*, or the creativity that relies on certain life experiences not shared by children. Thus, claims that children are *equally* creative seem hard to substantiate, and therefore compromise their share in the image of God. Conversely, if spontaneous creativity is the marker, then surely most adults are not fully human. The focus on vulnerability is even more concerning. Aside from the confusion over what is meant by vulnerability—whether it is simple openness to relationships or susceptibility to wounding specifically— it seems hard to posit this as the basis for an equal humanity, since children are more vulnerable to harm. In fact, whatever the capacity chosen, whether rationality, language ability, creativity, love, opposable thumbs, or the predilection for wearing plaid, there will always be humans who more or less live up to the ideal—and many humans who do not.

While I do not think it possible to come to a complete understanding of what it means to be the image of God—because both humans and God are mysteries—I propose that seeing the *imago Dei* in terms of intersubjectivity does the most justice to who humans are from birth to death as creatures created in the image of a Trinitarian God. By arguing this point, I hope to correct a trend in theology of children that remains bound to *a* capacity, like creativity, as the true marker of humanity. Under the auspices of intersubjectivity, we can understand freedom, language, love, self-transcendence, morality, rationality, and other capacities common to humans. Unlike a capacity-based approach, the question is not to what extent any human or group of humans lives up to the ideal capacity, but how human relationality makes possible a whole variety of abilities expressed in human life. Now, I am not suggesting that the biblical texts claim the image of God is intersubjectivity. Instead, I believe that the philosophical notion of intersubjectivity is the best tool we have right now for expressing and understanding what it means to be made in the image of God.

Intersubjectivity is the philosophical expression of our basic existence as neither a solipsistic being nor a social conglomerate; it emphasizes that our subjectivity is not just in relation with others but constituted by others.[41] Bernard Lonergan calls this "spontaneous intersubjectivity," which, while not eliminating our egoism, is the natural human orientation:

> Prior to the "we" that results from the mutual love of an "I" and a "thou," there is the earlier "we" that precedes the distinction of subjects and survives its oblivion. This prior "we" is vital and functional. Just as one spontaneously raises one's arm to ward off a blow against one's

head, so with the same spontaneity one reaches out to save another from falling. Perception, feeling, and bodily movement are involved, but the help given another is not deliberate but spontaneous. It is as if "we" were members of one another prior to our distinctions of each from the others.[42]

For Lonergan, spontaneous intersubjectivity is precognitive. His quote makes clear that this intersubjectivity is not the same thing as a predilection for interpersonal sociability; some people enjoy the company of others more, some less. But that personality trait, though dependent like all other traits on our intersubjective nature, is not what is meant by intersubjectivity. Paul Ricoeur embarks on a similar project in *Oneself as Another*, in which he writes about "a kind of otherness that is not (or not merely) the result of comparison is suggested by our title, otherness of a kind that can be constitutive of selfhood as such."[43] This intersubjectivity provides the foundation of our social bonds and our communities. What separates intersubjectivity from contractual accounts of human relationality is that intersubjectivity supposes a relationality internal to our subjectivity, as it were, and constitutive of it.

Philosophies of intersubjectivity begin not by considering the "complete" adult person, but by looking at the origins of human life; the parent-child relationship is central to notions of intersubjectivity.[44] We do not begin in blankness or neutrality, but are born into a matrix of beliefs, obligations, and relationships before we are aware of them. This intersubjectivity is constitutive of our subjectivity in a way that does not erase individuals but demonstrates their interconnectivity.[45] We should not imagine here the collective consciousness of fictive species like *Star Trek*'s Borg. Each person also knows themselves as an "I," knows that they have a personal existence and a history capable of being narrated. One source of the uniqueness of each individual is their body, though even in elements of bodily comportment, genetics, and mannerisms, they are indebted to those around them.[46] Their individuality exists within this account of intersubjectivity, this prior relationship with others.

By understanding humanity in terms of intersubjectivity, we can better appreciate that the child already *is* an intersubjective subject, not least through the ways in which infants, children, adolescents, and adults mutually impact each other. Infants are born into a world, a set of traditions, rituals, and obligations, that precedes their ability to recognize or question.[47] Parents and children mimic each other's expressions and movements and mirror each other's emotions.[48] The very presence of children changes their parents, as well as their wider communities. Children, by their very existence, as well as by their questions and actions, invite their parents to creatively reevaluate that which they will pass down.

Further, children open up a world of subjectivity that has been forgotten; children reveal to us aspects of our humanity. This happens even before a child is born: even before the face-to-face encounter there is the enfleshed, enwombed encounter of the mother and gestating child that invites the mother to reevaluate her view of and place in the world. Not only mothers do so, as is beautifully illustrated in the encounter between the main character, Theo, and a baby still inside his mother's womb in P.D. James's *Children of Men*. Theo is living a life of apathy in a time of state-sponsored narcissism following mass infertility. But when he encounters the child in Julian's womb, a child that is not even his, a feeling of awe washes over him. The baby's life opens to him new possibilities and brings new meaning. He is "freed for friendship, . . . love, . . . and faith" and begins from this moment to work for the good of others.[49] Even before they are born, children can teach us new values, new judgments, and new ways of being spontaneously intersubjective.[50]

Further, this account of humans as intersubjective subjects allows us to posit an asymmetry of relationship rather than one-way development between adult and child (and between adult and adolescent, adolescent and child, older child and younger child, toddler and infant, older adult and younger adult) that is predicated on a common humanity. This allows us to speak of the responsibilities adults have toward children, the limitations of childhood, and the development of capacities on a common foundation—unlike, for example, the Athenians, for whom both the wildness and purity of children was because they were like another species.[51] Similarly, it allows us to speak of the ways in which the goods of childhood, like creativity, humility, responsiveness to others, curiosity, resilience, aptitude for learning, and flexibility in turn call adults to see the world in new ways. In this asymmetry, each group contributes their own strengths to shared meaning-making and tasks.

Thus, intersubjectivity isn't simply another way of saying that children have generic value. Intersubjectivity tells us how children have value, and how they share in our humanity in general. It also tells us how they *already* communicate and share in the moral world. We find here the beginning of an idea of how children and adults can work together in relationship. Tied to the concept of intersubjectivity is the notion that we all have a drive toward knowledge and self-transcendence (I will talk about this more in the final section of this chapter and in future chapters). Our growth in language, desire, insight, and knowledge happens in the midst of—and is made possible by—our existence as intersubjective subjects. I will expand on this in the coming chapters in relation to children's moral agency and meaning-making around death and dying.

Understanding the *imago Dei* as intersubjectivity is foundational but not exhaustive. Intersubjectivity is not a capacity; it is not something that we have more or less of. It is, however, the foundation of all our capacities, including our capacity to love. But equally important is the idea that the *imago Dei* is never less than intersubjectivity, never less than the fact that our selves, unique as they are, are only made possible by relation with others and with God. We are intersubjective beings because we are children of God.

Intersubjectivity thus gives us a shared humanity that cannot be lost through the failure to exercise a certain capacity. From this foundation, we can confront concerns about what many theologians of children take to be the ambiguous attitude toward children found in historical theological texts and in the Bible. They find this ambiguous attitude because, while the biblical stories involving children are largely positive, children are also depicted as learning and developing, and as wild, immature, and sinful. But the fact that the Bible and Christian history have an ambiguous notion of children is not inherently a problem, unless this ambiguity extends to the conviction that children are less than human, or unless it is willfully blind to certain aspects of children's lives. In fact, this ambiguity is an appropriate rebuke to the view of childhood as innocent, sequestered, and priceless. Observation of the actual lives of children reveals that children can at times be unruly and even animal-like, as anyone who has trained an animal and raised a toddler knows. Many a child has eaten dirt and disobeyed their parents. Yet children also surprise us with their capacity for love, clarity of insight, and readiness to give and receive loyalty.

When Jesus sets the little child on his knee, he is not only calling on those around him to treat children with respect, he is raising up the child as a model of discipleship.[52] This reality is evoked powerfully by Jesus's words: "Truly I tell you, unless you change and become like little children, you will never enter the kingdom of heaven."[53] This child on Jesus's knee is not an abstract construction, but rather actual childhood is brought out in the mission of

Jesus, who deepens the significance of childhood by putting it in the context of the mission of the kingdom of God.[54] Child imagery is used throughout the New Testament (yes, including in Paul's letters!) to illustrate what it means for us to follow God, to be children of God. Children already know something of what it means to live as children of God.

But while children teach us, they are not valued for their instrumentality. God cares about the welfare of children. The treatment of orphans is held up throughout the Old Testament as the yardstick by which to measure Israel's conduct in the world. Parents were encouraged to raise their children and instruct them in the ways of God as part of their love for children. The psalmist tells us that this concern extends to the fetus; that God knows and cares for us even in the womb.[55] This extends even to children outside the covenant: God watches over and provides for Ishmael after he and his mother, Hagar, are cast out of Abraham's household.[56] Later, in Exodus, we are told of God's providential regard for Moses, who is found by the daughter of Pharaoh after being secreted in a basket by his mother. There are also, in both Testaments, multiple stories of children being raised from the dead. In 1 Kings, we read of the widow's son being resurrected, and in 2 Kings, Elisha performs a similar miracle, raising from the dead the son of a Shunammite woman.[57] In the New Testament, Jesus raises at least two children from the dead, casts out demons, and heals many others; children are not excluded from his healing ministry nor his promise of salvation.

Children, in their lack of self-sufficiency, help their seemingly self-reliant elders remember their creatureliness before God. Observing and recollecting childhood presents us "with an image of the relationship with God to which all humans are called."[58] Children stand as representative of humanity living between misery and grace, between the prior innocence and the hoped-for eschatology. Children, in their inquisitiveness and enthusiasm, illustrate "the divine blessing that underlies all human life, but which is generally overlaid by adult preoccupations."[59] All human beings—including children—have the capacity in human freedom to experience the divine self-communication.[60]

In other words, we do not become children of God only when we reach a particular stage of development; instead, human childhood is a double beginning: the beginning of an individual life in time, and the beginning of a life as a child of God. Children are already in a direct relationship with God. This is not to say that humans do not age and mature, but rather that maturity is not necessary for our experience of God. Children illustrate the incompleteness of all human beings before God, and model openness to God. In this way, childhood "is a basic condition which is always appropriate to a life that is lived aright."[61]

Importantly, our lasting childhood is not an idealized form of our "true selves," often expressed through ideas of our inner child (as Burman puts it, "the ideal version of ourselves that perhaps remains secret or carefully protected, that lies within us as something special or as yet unrealized potential"). Rahner's essay on childhood is short, and it is not always clear how he envisioned this childhood that is the goal of discipleship. But it is my position that there is no reclaiming of our fictional inner child, but rather our true self lies in our relationship to God as his children. Achieving this kind of childhood involves reclaiming certain forms of knowledge and ways of seeing the world that contradict dominant accounts of rationality. But it is not reclaiming some sinless proto-human time of innocence. A return to the child is not a return to the prelapsarian state inside ourselves, but rather a recognition that God's redemption is *already* at work in the life of a child. This view only makes sense rooted in a person's actual, lived childhood, not in a fantasy.

Finally, childhood is not a stage of life left behind, but extends into the eschaton. More than this, we can only understand childhood in light of this eschatological childhood.[62] As Rahner puts it,

> In the child a man begins who must undergo the wonderful adventure of remaining a child forever, becoming a child to an ever-increasing extent, making his childhood of God real and effective in this childhood of his, for this is the task of his maturity. It is only in the child that the child in the simple and absolute sense of the term really begins. And that is the dignity of the child, his task and his claim upon us all that we can and must help him in this task. In serving the child in this way, therefore, there can be no question of any petty sentimentality. Rather it is the eternal value and dignity of man, who must become a child, that we are concerned with, the man who only becomes a sharer in God's interior life in that he becomes that child which he only begins to be in his own childhood.[63]

That which is true eternally, that we are children of God, is lived out in the concrete here and now. But because all time is God's time, that which is lived out in the here and now continues into eternity.

Imagining this perpetual childhood can be a challenge; perhaps the closest we can come is in stories, such as MacDonald's story of the golden key I discussed above. We see ourselves in Mossy and Tangle, aging, journeying, maturing, and traveling through all life's stages. And perhaps we will be like Mossy and Tangle, who, on the other side of death, look youthful again and begin to climb the ladder into the heavens. One can only imagine that as they journey and "age" on the other side, they will become, like the Old Man of the Earth, a mere babe, wise beyond all others. And if they do, perhaps we will too.

✷✷✷

The implication of understanding the image of God as intersubjectivity, and of seeing the goal of human life as eternal childhood in God, is that we cannot flourish as human beings without children and childhood. We ought to name the aspects of childhood that model discipleship, value them in children, and seek to cultivate them in our lives. This is how we enter the second childhood that is wise, as Rahner puts it. Understanding these goods particular to childhood can help us begin to see how human beings of all ages have something to contribute to the shared human task of being God's children.

That children possess certain gifts when it comes to responding to God is illustrated in many biblical stories. In the Old Testament, the illustration of these gifts is often told in a story juxtaposing the faithfulness of a child against the faithlessness of adults. Samuel is a boy when he hears the voice of the Lord and his faithful response is in direct contrast with the actions of the High Priest Eli and his sons.[64] In a faithless nation, Isaiah hears and receives a specific call from God, and "the Davidic ruler described in [Isaiah] 11:1–5 will inaugurate an era in which children feature prominently."[65] Further, in contrast to the orphans who suffer from the injustice of Israel, Isaiah prophesies a child born to "us" who "will become the authoritative rule who embodies God's grace and peace."[66] Others, like Josiah and David, receive an indirect call from God through the actions of high priests Samuel and Hilkiah, respectively.[67]

That children possess certain gifts when it comes to a response to the word of God is demonstrated most strikingly by Jesus's words about children, when he says that we must become like little children in order to enter the kingdom of Heaven. "Jesus directly equates the reign of God with the least of these—with children—as the foundational rationale for receiving them."[68] I read this not as a generic attention to those who are the least in society, but as a particular referral to children. It is an invitation to see children as they are, rather than as they are not. In my view, the most beautiful part for readers of these biblical texts, and also of childhood studies, of philosophy of children, theology of children, and developmental psychology is the discovery of children's continual abilities to amaze, to ask new questions, to be far more capable than we give them credit for, to inspire a response.

These gifts arise from the fact that children, as intersubjective subjects, are self-transcendent. By this, I mean that they are teleologically oriented in their abundant and enthusiastic thirst for truth and goodness. In his endless desire for knowing, a child drives beyond his self, the self constituted by others, toward truth and goodness. He does this in and with others through his interpersonal relationships, his relationship to the world in its entirety, and in his relationship with God, who is truth and goodness. And yet, this drive beyond himself is at the same time highly personal and appropriated in the own operations of his knowing self.

Lonergan explores this human knowing through a non-exhaustive list of the everyday operations of human activity: "seeing, hearing, touching, smelling, tasting, inquiring, imagining, understanding, conceiving, formulating, reflection, marshalling and weighing the evidence, judging, deliberating, evaluating, deciding, speaking, writing."[69] These operations can be assigned to four levels of intentional consciousness found in all human knowing: experiencing, understanding, judging, and deciding. In response to a question like "what is it?" a human knower has an insight, a sudden grasp of how things are. But this is just an idea. In order to reach knowledge of the truth, he must ask himself "is it so?" He entertains questions for reflection: determining the conditions for truth and fulfilling them.[70]

So, for example, a child sees a bird on the lawn. She has a sudden insight: that is a Cooper's hawk. But this is only an idea, and she must question whether it is indeed the case, so she reflects: If it is truly a Cooper's hawk, what are the conditions to arrive at the judgment of fact? She can come up with a whole series of questions, such as whether these are common birds, whether they live in her area, what the identifying marks are, and the like. She answers these questions with a combination of observation, prior experience, and perhaps research. Once all these questions have been answered, she can know with a fair degree of certainty that this bird is a Cooper's hawk—this is what Lonergan calls arriving at a virtually unconditioned judgment. Sometimes arriving at this judgment of fact can be extremely swift, as habit and experience enable an ornithologist to but glance at a bird and correctly identify it. But other times, arriving at a judgment can be a lengthy process.

I will talk more in the coming chapters about how this self-transcendence plays out in relation to children's moral agency, but here I want to note two things. First, that all these operations of knowing are things that children *already* do. Second, while they clearly lack in some abilities, *children are better at some operations than adults.* I call these operations in which children excel the goods of childhood. What, then, are these goods of childhood that arise from our intersubjective and self-transcendent nature as children? It is impossible to write an exhaustive list, but I name imagination, wonder, loving dependency, imitation, and attention as some of these goods. In the following chapters, I will show how these goods are demonstrated in children's moral agency, and how they shape children's responses to death.

Children wonder. I mean this in the enchanted, enraptured sense where a child's whole body quivers with the delight of something new and unexpected. Think of when a child sees the moon in the daytime sky and stands watching it for ages. Or, equally, the way a child wonders at the shoe rack that moved location while they were at kindergarten, or at a smushed snail on the sidewalk. There exist romantic notions of children's wonderment in part because it is a phenomenon witnessed over and over again by parents, friends, families, and caregivers. "The child's enraptured sense of wonder in response to the parent's face, actions, and world train the parent to become more attentive to detail, more full of awe, and more awakened to a future that extends beyond the parent's own life through the life of the child."[71] Wonder can reshape the world.

This wonder is related to imagination, the ability to create new meanings and possibilities in any given place. Children do not divide the world into fact and fantasy but live in the interplay between the two. This allows them to hold on to a multiplicity of meaning that cannot be reduced to a simple, literal statement. Think of the way a child can be a princess-bear-fireman with no concern for contradiction. In this way, children can imagine themselves and the world to be other than it is. In their almost inexhaustible penchant for imaginative play, children create new ways of being in relation to self and other.[72] If we and the world around us are constituted by stories, as some theologians describe, then it is through the imagination that these stories develop and change.

Children excel at imitating and mirroring the attitudes, desires, and conduct of others.[73] This allows them to learn quickly in new relationships and surroundings.

The mirror can be uncomfortable sometimes. After spending significant time with her godmother, my daughter started to say, "Oh my gosh!" in a valley-girl style. Through this imitation, her godmother realized for the first time that she was in the habit of saying that. Children's excellence in imitation also gives them an advantage in learning from others: They soak up knowledge in an intimate, bodily sense rather than as a proposition that can be easily forgotten. This imitation and mirroring begins as pre-intentional, as young children are so attuned to others. We lose aspects of this attunement as we age.

Children are powerful observers. In fact, some elements of children's wondering and imitation, even imagination, may be due to this incredible ability to observe and interpret their surroundings. Children in nursery school have a keen grasp of the adults who come to pick up various children and can often distinguish each child's parents, grandparents, and other caregivers. Children who spend a significant amount of time in hospital settings have an intimate grasp of the hierarchy of the hospital staff, which jobs are performed by which type of staff person, and the rules and regulations not only pertaining to the children themselves, but to members of the hospital staff.[74] Because children, unlike adults, are much less likely to preselect the information that they consider relevant to any given task or circumstance, children outperform adults in task-irrelevant attention tests.[75] Adult attention is far more selective. This means that children see many things that adults miss.

Finally—and crucial for not only understanding what it means to be a child of God, but for understanding death and dying (as we will talk about in the latter sections of the book)—children do not experience dependency as a negative. In fact, children often revel in loving dependence. Think of the sheer joy on a baby or toddler's face when they see someone else, especially someone they recognize. Some children do this every time their parent looks at them. In this embrace of dependency especially, Elisabeth Kübler-Ross, famous for her depiction of the five stages of grief among the terminally ill, found much to learn from children. Many of the fears that adults have about losing control, about having to rely on others, are not shared by children, but embraced as something wonderful. Children not only need others, but they enjoy needing others. This dependency is constitutive of, not in violation to, their selfhood and dignity. This is, in part, why children are prone to spontaneous outbursts of affection. They are quick to love.

***

Who, then, is a child? A child is a young human being, best understood as falling between toddlerhood and puberty, a full sharer in our common humanity, created in the image of God, an intersubjective subject who is constituted by others and, crucially, a child of God. This account of humans as intersubjective subjects allows us to posit an asymmetry of relationship between adult and child that is predicated on a common humanity—both in the obligations adults have toward children, and the ways in which the goods of childhood call adults to see the world in new ways.

Childhood, then, is a relational term. What it means to be a child is understood in the context of what it means to be a child of God. It is understood in relation to childhood as it is lived out in the world, and to the goods of childhood. These goods of childhood do not mean that children are equally able to act in the world as adults, when by "equal" we mean alone and in existing social structures. But the goods of childhood call into question the idealization of adult abilities, upon which a stark and large divide between children and adults is predicated. This is why I am keen to keep a sense of development in our account of childhood. We have responsibilities toward children because of who they are, because of their increased vulnerability to harm and to poor teaching. But we have equally a responsibility to listen to them and to learn from them.

Children illuminate what it means to live as children of God. Children, in their lack of self-sufficiency, help their seemingly self-reliant elders remember their creatureliness before God. Further, childhood itself already participates in God, and is not something left behind in maturity, but is something that endures eschatologically. We do not become children of God only when we reach a particular stage of development. Instead, human childhood is a double beginning: the beginning of an individual life in time, and the beginning of a life as a child of God.

NOTES

1 Edmund Newey, *Children of God: The Child as Source of Theological Anthropology* (Burlington: Ashgate, 2012), 61–62.
2 Heather Montgomery, *An Introduction to Childhood: Anthropological Perspectives on Children's Lives* (Chichester: Wiley-Blackwell, 2009), 50.
3 Montgomery, *Introduction to Childhood*, 204–207.
4 Michael Wyness, "Children's Participation: Definitions, Narratives and Disputes" in *Theorising Childhood: Citizenship, Rights and Participation*, eds. Claudio Baraldi and Tom Cockburn (London: Palgrave MacMillan, 2018), 59. See also the introduction.

5   See Erica Burman, *Deconstructing Developmental Psychology*, 3rd ed. (London: Routledge, 2017), 14–30.

6   Montgomery, *Introduction to Childhood*, 144, 146–147.

7   Replicated recently in *The Economist* Childhood: Special Reports, January 5, 2019.

8   Paul Bloom, *Just Babies: The Origins of Good and Evil* (New York: Random House, 2013), especially 7–32.

9   Burman, *Deconstructing Developmental Psychology*, ix–xii.

10 Montgomery, *Introduction to Childhood*, 50.

11 Bonnie Miller-McLemore, "Children's Voices, Spirituality, and Mature Faith" in *Children's Voices: Children's Perspectives in Ethics, Theology and Religious Education*, eds. Annemie Dillen and Didier Pollefeyt (Leuven: Uitgeverij Peeters, 2010), 19.

12 Burman, *Deconstructing Developmental Psychology*, ix–xii. "Yet national political discourse seems to have increasingly intensified its focus on the regulation of parenting, and especially mothering, making mothers quasi-entrepreneurs in preparing their children for the market while at the same time being sold a form of 'cruel optimism' that overstates not only parenting agency but also responsibility."

13 Edmund Newey, *Children of God: The Child as Source of Theological Anthropology* (Burlington: Ashgate, 2012), 61–2.

14 Newey, *Children of God*, 7, 61.

15 Nicholas Orme, *Medieval Children* (New Haven: Yale University Press, 2001) 27–30 on baptism, 321–328 on children and the law; Mark Golden, *Children and Childhood in Classical Athens*, 2nd ed. (Baltimore: Johns Hopkins University Press, 2015), 2.

16 Montgomery, *Introduction to Childhood*, 19.

17 Jaclyn Duffin, *History of Medicine: A Scandalously Short Introduction*, 2nd ed. (Toronto: University of Toronto Press, 2010), 361.

18 See Duffin, 369–70; The answer to whether this experimentation has stopped largely depends on one's definition of medical experimentation. One key difference is now that the enrollment of children in clinical trials requires the informed consent of parents or caregivers and, in theory, must meet the criteria for "best interests."

19 Duffin, *History of Medicine*, 352. See also Orme, *Medieval Children*, 95–6.

20 Bruno Vanobbergen, "The Disappearing Child or the Disappearing Adult? On the Image of the Innocent Child in a Commercialised Childhood," in *Children's Voices: Children's Perspectives in Ethics, Theology and Religious Education*, eds. Annemie Dillen and Didier Pollefeyt (Leuven: Uitgeverij Peeters, 2010), 166.

21 Burman, *Deconstructing Developmental Psychology*, 9

22 See, for example, John Wall, *Ethics in the Light of Childhood* (Washington, DC: Georgetown University Press, 2010), Chapter 1 "Three Enduring Models," 13–32; Hugh Pyper, "Children," in *The Oxford Companion to Christian Thought*, ed. Adrian Hastings (Oxford: Oxford University Press, 2000), 100; David Jensen, *Graced Vulnerability*, 11. Miller-McLermore, *Let the Children Come*, 1.

23 Marcia J. Bunge, "Introduction," in *The Child in the Bible*, ed. Marcia J. Bunge (Grand Rapids: Eerdmans, 2008), 16–7; Patrick McKinley Brennan, "Introduction" in *The Vocation of the Child*, ed. Patrick McKinley Brennan (Grand Rapids: Eerdmans, 2008), 221–223.

24 Bonnie J. Miller-McLemore, *Let the Children Come: Reimagining Childhood from a Christian Perspective* (San Francisco: Jossey-Bass, 2003), 89.

25 Miller-McLemore, 90; Joyce Ann Mercer, *Welcoming Children: A Practical Theology of Childhood* (St. Louis: Chalice Press, 2005), 73–76.

26 Harry Adams, *Justice for Children: Autonomy Development and the State* (Albany: State University of New York Press, 2007), 18–19.

27 Miller-McLemore, *Let the Children Come*, 91.

28 Karen-Marie Yust, "God is *Not* Your Divine Butler and Therapist! Countering 'Moralistic Therapeutic Deism' by Teaching Children the Art of Theological Reflection," in *Children's Voices: Children's Perspectives in Ethics, Theology and Religious Education*, eds. Annemie Dillen and Didier Pollefeyt (Leuven: Uitgeverij Peeters, 2010), 55.

29 Montgomery, *Introduction to Childhood*, 23–24.

30 WHO, *Children are not little adults*, http://www.who.int/ceh/capacity/Children_are_ not_little_adults.pdf. See also Burman *Deconstructing Developmental Psychology*, 67–86.

31 See Canada, for example. Some federal laws against child pornography apply to material involving children, with children being those under the age of eighteen, whereas under the Youth Criminal Justice Act, child "means a person who is or, in the absence of evidence to the contrary, appears to be less than twelve years old." This act distinguishes between a child and a young person, which "means a person who is or, in the absence of evidence to the contrary, appears to be twelve years old or older, but less than eighteen years old." Ontario, Manitoba, Quebec, Alberta, and Prince Edward Island define a minor child as a person under the age of eighteen. The remaining provinces and territories define a minor child as one under nineteen years of age, with the exception of Newfoundland, which differentiates between a minor (age sixteen and under) and a youth (ages sixteen to eighteen). For some of these provinces, however, the age at which a person is legally considered a minor is different from the definition of a minor for the purposes of child protection: Ontario, Nova Scotia, New Brunswick, and the territories set the age for child protection as sixteen. From https://tinyurl.com/2p9xwfan.

32 Julie Faith Parker, *Valuable and Vulnerable: Children in the Hebrew Bible, Especially the Elisha Cycle* (Providence: Brown University, 2013), 41–74.

33 Golden, *Children and Childhood in Classical Athens*, 2, 11. See also Cornelia B. Horn, and John W. Martens, *"let the little children come to me": Childhood and Children in Early Christianity* (Washington, DC: The Catholic University of America Press, 2009), 6–16.

34 Miller-McLemore, "Children's Voices," 46.

35 George MacDonald, "The Golden Key," in *The Complete Fairy Tales*, ed. U. C Knoepflmacher (New York: Penguin Books, 1999), 120–144.

36 See the Genesis text. See also Terrence E. Fretheim, " 'God was with the boy' (Genesis 21:20): Children in the Book of Genesis," in *The Child in the Bible*, ed. Marcia J. Bunge (Grand Rapids: Eerdmans, 2008), 4, 6–7.

37 Fretheim, 9; Miller-McLemore, *Let the Children Come*, 93.

38 Sibley Towner, "Children and the Image of God," in *The Child in the Bible*, ed. Marcia J. Bunge (Grand Rapids: Eerdmans, 2008), 313–321.

39 Towner, "Children and the Image of God," 309–310.

40 See John Wall, *Ethics in the Light of Childhood* and David H. Jensen, *Graced Vulnerability: A Theology of Childhood* (Cleveland: Pilgrim Press, 2005), as two examples.

41 In this understanding of intersubjectivity, I draw on Paul Ricoeur, Bernard Lonergan, and on Brock Bahler's project *Childlike Peace in Merleau-Ponty and Levinas:*

Intersubjectivity as Dialectical Spiral, which draws on Merleau-Ponty and Levinas and develops the centrality of the parent-child relationship for understanding intersubjectivity. Paul Ricoeur, *Oneself as Another*, trans. Kathleen Blamey (Chicago: University of Chicago Press, 1992); Bernard Lonergan, *Method in Theology* (Toronto: University of Toronto Press, 1990); Bernard Lonergan, *Insight*, vol 3, *The Collected Works of Bernard Lonergan* (Toronto: University of Toronto Press, 1988); Brock Bahler, *Childlike Peace in Merleau-Ponty and Levinas: Intersubjectivity as Dialectical Spiral* (New York: Lexington Books, 2016).

42 Lonergan, *Method*, 57; Ricoeur, *Oneself as Another*, 3.

43 Paul Ricoeur, *Oneself as Another*, trans. Kathleen Blamey (Chicago: University of Chicago Press, 1992), 3.

44 See especially Brock Bahler's *Childlike Peace.*

45 Bahler, *Childlike Peace*, x; Ricoeur, *Oneself as Another*, 1–26.

46 Bahler, *Childlike Peace*, 7.

47 Bahler, 20.

48 Gandolfo, *Power and Vulnerability*, 47–59; For example, though pre-linguistic and sometimes even characterized as precognitive, "the infant assumes a latent meaning in the actions of others, is "capable of the same intentions," and responds by imitating their gestures, facial features, and so on." Bahler, *Childlike Peace*, 38. Balthasar puts it this way: even in the womb, the child is already other. Hans Urs von Balthasar, *Unless You Become Like This Child*, trans. Erasmo Leiva-Merikakis (San Francisco: Ignatius Press, 1991), 16.

49 Craig E. Mattson and Virginia LaGrand, "Eros at the World's End: Apocalyptic Attention in the Love Stories of Graham Greene and P. D. James," *Renascence* 64 (2912): 286.

50 Mark T. Miller, *The Quest for God and the Good Life: Lonergan's Theological Anthropology* (Washington, DC: Catholic University of America Press, 2013), 79; Bahler, *Childlike Peace*, x.

51 Cf. Mark Golden, *Children and Childhood in Classical Athens*, 2, and my discussion in chapter 1.

52 In the gospel accounts, but especially in the book of John, child imagery is closely linked to an identity: the disciples and followers of Jesus as children of God. James M. M. Francis, *Adults as Children: Images of Childhood in the Ancient World and the New Testament* (New York: Peter Lang, 2006), 162–6.

53 Matthew 18:2–4.

54 Francis, *Adults as Children*, 147.

55 Psalm 139; This concern is also illustrated in the Levitical laws, in which are found rules about having children, sacrifices after childbirth, waiting periods after childbirth, penalties for striking a pregnant woman and causing her to lose the child. See Kristine Henriksen Garroway, *Growing up in Ancient Israel: Children in Material Culture and Biblical Texts* (Atlanta: SBL Press, 2018).

56 Fretheim, "God was with the boy," 12–13; Cf. Genesis 17. This story is notable because it specifically depicts God hearing the cry of a child: God hears the cry of Ishmael, and makes a promise to him.

57 1 Kings 17:21–2 "Then he stretched himself out on the boy three times and cried out to the Lord, "Lord my God, let this boy's life return to him!" The Lord heard Elijah's cry, and the boy's life returned to him, and he lived." See also 2 Kings 4.

58 Newey, *Children of God*, 34. Newey finds this approach taken in the theology of Thomas Traherne. Cf. Thomas Traherne, *The Works of Thomas Traherne: Vol 1*, ed. Jan Ross (Cambridge: D. S. Brewer, 2005), 440–445.

59 Newey, *Children of God*, 35.

60 Mercer, *Welcoming Children*, 150

61 Karl Rahner, "Ideas for a Theology of Childhood," in *Theological Investigations Vol. 8: Further Theology of the Spiritual Life 2*, trans. David Bourke (New York: Herder and Herder, 1971), 47.

62 Newey, *Children of God*, 19, 93; Rahner, "Ideas," 35–36.

63 Rahner, "Ideas," 50.

64 1 Samuel 3.

65 Lapsley, "Look," 88–90. Isaiah, notable as perhaps Israel's most important prophet, and proclaimer of the future Messiah, was most likely a young child when God first called him to prophecy. Children also feature prominently in the book of Isaiah in his "focus on orphans, and way Israel itself is described metaphorically as a child in the book." Jaqueline E. Lapsley, "Look! The Children and I Are as Signs and Portents in Israel": Children in Isaiah," in *The Child in the Bible*, ed. Marcia J. Bunge (Grand Rapids: Eerdmans, 2008); 82.

66 Lapsley, "Look," 88–90.

67 2 Chronicles 34. Josiah was only eight years old when he became King of Judah, and his actions of reform are set in contrast to the actions of his father, Amon, who did evil in the sight of the Lord and was assassinated by his household servants.

68 Miller-McLemore, *Let the Children Come*, 95; Francis, *Adults as Children*, 146.

69 Lonergan, *Method*, 9.

70 See Bernard Lonergan, *Insight*, vol. 3, *The Collected Works of Bernard Lonergan* (Toronto: University of Toronto Press, 1988), 296–340.

71 Bahler, *Childlike Peace*, 34.

72 Wall, *Ethics*, 51.

73 See Paul Bloom *Just Babies* and Brock Bahler *Childlike Peace*.

74 Myra Bluebond-Langner, *The Private Worlds of Dying Children* (Princeton: Princeton University Press, 1980), 135–165.

75 D. J. Plebanek and V. M. Sloutsky, "Costs of Selective Attention: When Children Notice What Adults Miss," *Psychological Science,* 28 (2017): 723–732.

CHAPTER 2

Can a Child Live a Good Life?

In the previous chapter, I argued that children share fully in humanity, and thus what we say about theological anthropology must include children. Children are not *other* but fully human, made in the image of God, and part of our eschatological future. The goal of the Christian life is to become like children, and we learn how to do this through our own childhoods: lived, observed, and recollected. Children are already made in the image of God, and already in relationship with God. When Jesus set a child on his knee and declared that we must become children to enter the kingdom of God, he was not expressing a romantic notion of childhood innocence. Instead, he was making a profound statement about what it means to be human.

However, simply acknowledging the shared humanity of children does not pay sufficient attention to their moral lives. We must go a step further, and recognize that because children are human beings, they are therefore moral beings. This understanding requires us to rethink fundamental aspects of human moral nature, much in the same way that recognizing the inclusion of women, people of color, and people with disabilities has prompted a reconsideration of what it means to be human. This chapter presents an account of the moral agency of children, building on the understanding of children as intersubjective and self-transcending subjects introduced in the previous chapter.

This chapter asks the question "Can a child live a good life?" rather than "Can a child make moral decisions?" because while decision-making is an important aspect of morality, it is not the only, and not even the most important. Attending to children's moral lives is a potent reminder that moral agency is not simply, or even predominantly, about a certain denuded rationalist type of *thinking and deciding*, nor is it limited to specific moral issues. By focusing on what it means to live according to that which is *good*, and by expanding our understanding of moral subjectivity and moral agency, we can see the many ways children already live in relation to goodness, seek the good, and reveal goodness to those around them.

Because children seek the good, and because they are intersubjective and self-transcendent subjects, children can also fruitfully deliberate, make decisions, and act morally. As I will explain in this chapter, they are genuine moral subjects and agents. This agency is grounded in children's ability to seek the good, to make meaning, to act, to imitate, to use language creatively, to grasp a plurality of meaning, to reach judgments, to contribute to the meaning of others and shape their understanding. It is grounded in intersubjective subjectivity, and it is grounded in a particular story: where subjectivity, agency, and wholeness are found in the Trinitarian God in whose image we are made.

As proper moral agents, children should share in moral decision-making, particularly when they are the ones most affected by certain decisions. This chapter will set the stage for a more specific discussion about children's place in end-of-life decision-making in chapter 5. Here, I will situate decision-making in a broader framework in which children are our partners in the shared human effort to seek and love that which is good. A comprehensive account of what it means for children to seek the good will have to be another project.

Children are moral subjects and agents because they live in relation to God as images and as children of God. Following the logic of the previous chapter, this chapter considers the moral lives of actual children, as well as the moral goals of eternal childhood in God. This will require us to think about moral agency in a different way—not in terms of an idealized (wealthy, independent, male) adult agent, but in terms of *how moral selfhood and agency begins*. It begins, like human life itself, in relationship to others and God. We can explore these beginnings through recollecting our own childhood, by observing children in real life and in story, and especially by engaging with children in moral exploration.

Children are also moral agents because they are subjects, subjects who engage already at a young age in the structure of human knowing and arrive already at judgments of fact and value. Children learn from adults, and they have limitations, but these do not put them in a separate moral world and are not on account of a different humanity. Moreover, children bring unique gifts to the moral realm and challenge adult understandings. They are exemplars of the desire to know, and of what it means to be children of God. This account of moral subjectivity and agency provides space for understanding the influence of others, of formation, of language, of imagination, and of imitation in the moral life.

Children respond in moral ways, make moral meaning, choose moral actions, and develop moral character. Yet they are not cognitively or morally identical to adults. Children have particular gifts they bring in the drive for knowledge of the good. It is our task as adults to recognize and nurture these abilities. In their (often spontaneous) response to others, children call us to respond to their presence, actions, questions, and opinions, which can reveal to us the narrowness of our own moral deliberations. At the same time, children need guidance, accommodation, and help. Just because children are genuine moral agents does not mean they are equally responsible. Thus, recent efforts to increase children's participation in moral decision-making by simply extending the right to decide to younger and younger children fail to properly support or protect children. In our mutual but asymmetrical relationship, attending to children reveals that *shared* decision-making starts with our entanglement with others instead of individual autonomy.

But so far, this discussion says little about what this moral selfhood and agency looks like in practice. It risks romanticism. Children are not pure and innocent actors who exist in a quasi-spiritual state of enlightenment, angelic proto-humans who sagely advise us. They are flawed and sinful too. They are capable of doing the right thing, and also of doing wrong. They need to grow and develop in their love and knowledge of the good. But as I explained in the previous chapter, the idea of intersubjectivity lets us fruitfully discuss development without worrying about dehumanization. Children are genuine moral agents, but they are also moral agents in development. Attending to them reminds us that adults, too, are moral agents in development. Similarly, by understanding that children bring particular gifts to our humanity and that they represent the goal of discipleship, we can talk about development without implying that its ultimate goal is an idealized adult individualist agency. So, in the following sections, I will consider how children develop morally, what teaching and guidance they require, and what gifts they bring to the moral development of their seniors.

***

A child is a moral subject or moral self because she is an intersubjective and self-transcending subject who seeks the good. She is born into a human community constituted by spontaneous intersubjectivity and by common meaning. That is, she is born into a community that already seeks the good, uses moral language, and creates moral meaning. She participates in the same moral world as her community even before she is aware that this community (or morality itself) exists. Children thus begin life in embodied relationship with other moral subjects and agents. Their subjectivity arises from this "we" and their presence awakens transformative love, new communicative acts of meaning, and new possibilities. And children can already achieve what is most important in the moral life, even as they continue to grow in reason, language, and virtue, for they are capable of loving God. Children live in relationship to God, who is good.

Moral subjectivity and moral agency presuppose each other. In the human being, the two are indistinct: We are moral subjects because we are agents, and agents because we are subjects. Because of this, there is no clean line between moral subjectivity and agency; they can be separated only in reflection, not in lived experience. Thus, when I talk about the moral subject in this section, I will inevitably be talking about the moral agent too. I separate the two in this reflection, however, because moral selfhood is so frequently forgotten. By moral selfhood, I mean to talk about who a person *is* and how they flourish.

I begin here because moral agency is so tightly linked in the cultural imagination to decision and action, and this bias is repeated in psychological studies of children's morality, which focus on their individual ability to decide and act. Thus, to talk about moral agency is to talk primarily about action. This is not an inherent problem. But it is at least a problem of communication because the moral life does not begin in discrete acts stemming from rational deliberation, but in mutual feeling and desire. This mutuality is the spontaneous intersubjectivity I described in the previous chapter, which supposes a relationality that is both internal to our subjectivity and constitutive of it. Intersubjectivity thus goes hand in hand with sensitivity, our spontaneous feelings that are in some way natural to us, though since these two things are both precritical, parsing the difference between them is not possible. In other words, our spontaneous desires and feelings are both natural and habituated.[1] But even what is natural to us, our bodies and desires, are received from others. This means that our starting point is one of reception. We *receive* the moral life rather than create it.

Reception does not mean determinism. A child receives her moral world from others but integral to her own moral selfhood is her personal reflection on inherited and communal values.[2] The ability to question and make decisions about the things they receive is also an important part of children's development, including their moral development, and we expect a different level of responsibility from toddlers, children, and adolescents on this basis. It is this ability to reflect on what we are doing, and to make our own choices, that allows us to reject what we have been taught, to leave oppressive situations, and to recognize the insufficiency or wrongness of values that we have received.[3] All children are, like us, their own person from infancy. Even though it is not possible to draw eternal and perfect boundaries between the self and other, it is still an important distinction, rooted in our unique access to ourselves, our ability to know ourselves as an "I," to narrate our life story, and to know ourselves as responsible agents of action. The uniqueness of the individual is precious, when held in tension with the communal and social nature of all people.

As her own person, the child is a moral subject, constituted by others and seeking truth and goodness in her conscious and ethical intentionality. In the previous chapter, I described the operations of conscious intentionality named by Bernard Lonergan and argued that these were all activities children already *do*, if not on the same level as adults. In fact, for Lonergan, children are the exemplar of the human desire to know. Children see, hear, touch, taste. They inquire, imagine, understand, conceive, formulate. They reflect, they marshal and weigh evidence, they judge, deliberate, evaluate, decide, speak, and (usually once they reach school age) write. They are rational, using at least four tools of nonformal reason: observation, formal and informal reasoning methods, creative construction, and systematic critical assessment.[4]

This intentionality suggests an account of rationality much broader than that of inductive or deductive reasoning, unfolding across Lonergan's four levels of intentional consciousness:

There is the *empirical* level on which we sense, perceive, imagine, feel, speak, move. There is an *intellectual* level on which we inquire, come to understand, express what we have understood, work out the presuppositions and implications of our expression. There is the *rational* level on which we reflect, marshal evidence, pass judgment on the truth or falsity, certainty, or probability, of a statement. There is the *responsible* level on which we are concerned with ourselves, our own operations, our goals, and so deliberate about possible courses of action, evaluate them, decide, carry out our decisions.[5]

These four levels are not progressive throughout a person's life, but rather "in everyday, commonsense performance, all four levels are employed continuously without any explicit distinction between them."[6] They are part of every human, including children, even if some operations are only partially expressed. And they are grounded in the unrestricted desire for truth and goodness.[7]

Following Lonergan's account of conscious intentionality, Patrick Byrne developed a theory of ethical intentionality, where he posits a "compound structure of . . . knowing and doing" that he calls "the structure of ethical intentionality."[8] This structure has thinking, feeling, deciding, and acting in dynamic relationship to each other, and in relationship to all the operations of conscious intentionality, since proper ethical deliberation must include a proper account of the situation and possible responses. To the list of cognitive operations (like seeing, smelling, inquiring, imagining, and reflecting), Byrne adds activities pertaining to ethical intentionality: "feeling, practical inquiring, practical insight, value inquiring, value reflecting, reflective understanding of value, value judging, deliberating, choosing/deciding, and acting."[9] These activities, too, are intrinsically and dynamically related. That is, these activities occur together in practice and are only separable upon reflection.

Like Lonergan's operations, all these operations that Byrne names are *already* performed by children. Children feel (how they feel!), they inquire, they value, they reflect, they act. If children are the exemplar of the human desire to know, here they are also exemplars of the human desire to be good. We see this in, among other things, their enthusiastic and spontaneous response to others, imaginative solutions to problems, generosity with self and possessions, and constant "why" questions about moral categories and ideas. We witness these operations in the lives of children around us and see them reflected in stories about children. After his adventures with North Wind, Diamond engages curiously with the world, responding to others, reasoning about his surroundings, making judgments, and seeking to ameliorate the lives of others.

Feelings are integral to this account of ethical intentionality, because feelings are apprehensions of value or disvalue—that is, of what is good. This means that valuing is not simply a function of cognitive assent to a theoretical notion of what is good. Instead, it echoes in our bodies, in the desire to be close to that which we determine to be good. Researchers have found this to be true even in babies of a few months old. Witnessing two people, one who helps another with a task, and one who hinders, infants demonstrate a clear preference to pay attention to and be near the helper.[10] Contrary to ethical theories that dismiss children's powerful affective responses as inhibitions to proper moral thought and action, here feelings are integral to morality. This is not to say that children are morally perfect. Feelings, like thoughts, need to be trained and nurtured to seek that which is good in line with the entirety of one's moral selfhood. But children's spontaneous affective responses are part of genuine moral subjectivity.

It is specifically his affective response to others, heightened after his visit to the world at North Wind's back, that drives Diamond's moral actions and reasoning in MacDonald's story. Diamond's concern about his parents' well-being, especially after his father loses his job and becomes ill, pushes him to learn to harness a horse and drive a London cab. He sings to his mother and entertains his baby brother, activities that bring joy to himself as well. Because his actions spring from a well of love, he is not preoccupied with his own problems, but has compassion to spare. His concern about the ill street-sweeper, Nanny, leads him to enlist the help of a man he barely knows, but judges to be good. This friendship with Mr. Raymond eventually sees Diamond's family and Nanny well taken care of by the time Diamond dies. His feelings are not separate from his moral response, but part and parcel of it, intimately related to his experiencing, understanding, reasoning, and judging.

This account of conscious and ethical intentionality, which is developmental, differs from Lockean and evolutionary accounts of moral development because it does not view its stages as tied to specific biological capacities, nor as *progressive*. That is, we do not start life in only experience or feeling, then add the intellectual, then the rational, and finally the responsible. Instead, these four levels function continuously, and the operations are performed concurrently. But while this development is not progressive, it is *patterned*. Our experience of the world is not pure; we cannot see and hear everything "as it is." What we experience is patterned by what we understand, know, and do, which in turn is determined by the meanings we have inherited and create. This patterning is what allows us to, for example, pick out a friend's voice in the din of a crowded bar. But this patterning also shapes our response, including our affective response, to moral situations.

This structure of ethical intentionality relies on the existence of others. That is, when approaching most situations, there is already a trove of knowledge from those who have come before on which we can draw.[11] These operations of ethical intentionality can also be shared through communicative acts of meaning. For example, a child can experience something as fair or unfair because she has received categories for judgment from someone else, or because someone else has modeled reasoning about fairness to her. Individuals are not only constituted by others, but live in community where judgments, acts, concepts, and past experiences are shared communicatively between members. Thus, we can meaningfully speak of the individual intentional consciousness (I can know myself as an *I*), but in actuality, any given individual lives in a shared world. If, as Brock Bahler thinks, an infant can share the intentionality of her parents, then her experiences are already patterned by the consciousness of others.[12] This is why Lonergan is mistaken, I believe, when he describes the first few months of life as existing in the "realm of pure experience."[13]

Readers familiar with Lonergan and Byrne's work may think them a strange choice for a moral theology of children. The structure of ethical intentionality Byrne envisions is more complex and demanding than many ethical theories. To know and do good requires common sense combined with scientific theoretical knowledge; it involves deep knowledge of a situation, the ability to imagine and weigh the possible and probable consequences of a course of actions, and a grasp of what is truly of value. It requires moral and cognitive conversion, so that our thoughts and feelings align with that which is true and good. To arrive at proper judgment, we must ask and answer all the relevant questions.

But in my work, this complexity is not the problem it appears to be. I am not arguing that children are, by themselves, full, responsible, ethical agents. Instead, I am arguing that children are *genuine moral agents who engage in the same structure of ethical intentionality* as every other human being. Not only that, but at times they engage in it better than adults through their unbiased questions and spontaneous responses to others. Byrne's account makes clear that there is no perfect, static adult agency that is achieved when we reach the pinnacle of our biological capacities. It does not allow us to use one criterion, like brain plasticity, as the marker of moral capability. There is no transition point from proto-ethical to ethical; this dynamic structure is continuous in the human ethical intentionality. The formation of ethical intentionality in childhood continues in us throughout our whole lives, as our experiences, knowledge, and feelings are patterned and developed, and as we appropriate ourselves as those who, from infancy, seek and do the good in an integrated way.

Childhood is not a discrete stage of life but continues through our existence. This is true not only for theology of children, but for moral theology as well. Ethical intentionality—the experiences, judgments, reasonings, and understandings we receive and create from our infancy—continues through our lives. What does this mean in practice? Here the work of philosopher Gareth Matthews is helpful. Against theories of *concept replacement*, common in many developmental accounts, Matthews argues for *concept maturation*. Matthews describes five elements of moral development: paradigms, defining characteristics, range of cases, adjudication of conflicting moral claims, and moral imagination. As we age, we will mature and occasionally even transform these five elements, but the ideas, concepts, and actions that form our childhood continue to operate in us as adolescents, adults, and into old age.

For example, a young child may understand the concept of lying through the paradigm of saying they did not do something in order to escape punishment, or in a more general way as saying something is false when they know it to be true. They may draw on defining characteristics of what is (and is not) lying by appealing to various cases in which they thought something was a lie, and by considering conflicts such as whether lying to protect a friend is a good or bad thing, or even a lie at all. They can imagine different responses to moral conflict, like whether lying is the proper response to a lie, or whether there is a potion that would make lies glow in the air. They may engage imaginatively with whether telling a lie changes their bodies or even who they are, as in the story of Pinocchio's nose.

Ideally, as children expand their experience in the world, these paradigms will expand, mature, and perhaps even be transformed. Children will imagine new responses to situations as they encounter them. Of course, for many of us, these childhood paradigms continue into adulthood unquestioned. Many adults make individual and political decisions that are colored by simplistic ideas about lying, even in the face of evidence that defining the characteristics of a lie is extremely difficult. And when we adults do engage with these paradigms, consider various definitions, and adjudicate whether a given situation can be characterized as a lie, we must note that we do so in the same manner as children. Children live in ethical worlds that are structured in exactly the same way ours are; their views are thus communicative with ours.

It is also worth noticing that paradigms, cases, definitions, and adjudications do not only emerge from a child's reflection but are *given* by others. Think about how a child learns what a lie is. When she lies, the adults (and other children) around her name the action as a lie. They may provide an explanation of why that action is a lie, why lies are wrong, and why other actions that seem similar are not lies. When a parent divides a cookie, he gives one equal part to each child and, when questioned, often explains that this is the fair way to divide the cookie. In this way, he is communicating a notion of fairness, and a child experiences the feeling and concept of fairness. This is part of what I mean when I say that our moral worlds are received from others. From the beginning, the operations of the moral subject are patterned by the communicative actions of others, through their words, expressions, actions, and very bodies.

A child's reasoning and judgment is not only formed through the reasoning and judgment of others but is also conditioned by her surroundings. We can think about the example of Naaman and his slave girl in 2 Kings 5.[14] The little servant girl, described thus in juxtaposition to her master, "a big man," fulfills her responsibilities to her master and to God when she tells Naaman how to seek healing for his leprosy. Her role in the story comprises only one or two verses. But with this little information, we can picture a child who is triply vulnerable on account of her gender, her role as servant, and her identity as a spoil of war. But on hearing about her master's illness, she offers a caring response. She recalls that there is a prophet and remembers where to find him. She also demonstrates her faith: She says that if her master visits the prophet, he will be healed. If we think of this according to Lonergan's and Matthews's schemes, we can interpret the story like this: The servant girl experiences (hears or sees) her master's illness. She understands the cause of the illness and reasons about possible responses. She recalls the prophet and his power. She is moved by Naaman's situation and acts. Perhaps she understands her own role according to the paradigm of service to her master, or of love of her neighbor. Her act is only one small part of the story, and it is Elijah who heals Naaman. But it is the little servant girl who sets him on that path.

Still, even as an ethicist who focuses on children, I can struggle to think of a child as a moral subject in a real, rather than proto-moral, sense. I find myself repeatedly influenced by the pervasive image of the moral subject as the *autonomous* subject. Autonomy is not value-free but contains normative ideals of what it means to be human.[15] This chapter is not the place to engage deeply with the centrality of autonomy in Western post-Enlightenment culture, nor, sadly, with the fascinating and complex philosophical notions of autonomy. Instead, drawing especially on insights from feminist and disability thinkers, I will limit myself to discussing a few general elements of the cultural ideal of autonomous moral subjectivity that has led to the conclusion that children are, at best, proto-moral subjects and agents.

These symbolic notions of autonomy operate powerfully in the public imagination. They are tied up with the ideal of libertarian theory: the rugged male individualist, a rational, maximizing chooser.[16] This autonomous subject is an abstract and disinterested thinker who arrives at moral conclusions through objective, rational deliberation. That this conception of autonomy is not presented in many theoretical works makes it more dangerous—it colors our imaginations in a way that is unexplicit and therefore not subject to critical evaluation. This hyperbolized view of autonomy pervades society, and its image of independence and power is seductive and surprisingly resistant to critique.[17]

Centrally, this normative vision of what a person should be excludes children as well as people with disabilities, women, those facing economic or other kinds of oppression, and (usually) the elderly. It is a vision of human personhood at odds with childhood, and with what it means to be children of God. This vision posits that we are independent and self-made, and that we can live without restraint or limitation from outside influence and from our own inclinations. It claims that our dignity is dependent on our rationality. Though this model of autonomy seductively claims that humans are characterized by equality, this equality is predicated on a narrow vision of humanity: the healthy adult male.

Harry Adams's *Justice for Children* is a remarkable example of how this model influences the exclusion of children from the moral realm. His book lays out legal and moral grounds for intervening in the care of children who are being prevented from reaching their highest potential autonomy. In his quest to protect children, however, Adams ends up devaluing them. In his scheme, children are valuable not as children, but for what they will one day become. He introduces a scale of six "autonomy levels" ranging from 0 to 5, where 0 is fully nonautonomous, 5 is fully autonomous, and 3 is the minimal level of autonomy necessary for self-governance.[18] Children fall somewhere between 0 and 2, depending on their stage of development, though Adams does acknowledge that some older adolescents can meet the criteria of 3.

That children do not meet his qualifications for autonomy is much less worrying than how he talks about those in the lower levels. Those with autonomy "lead an active, dignified and contemplative human life," as opposed to those who are nonautonomous, who lead a "merely passive and unreflective animal-like existence."[19] He goes as far as to say, "Surely a life without autonomy is grossly subpar, if not in some ways subhuman."[20] While Adams does acknowledge that there are valuable traits other than autonomy, the dehumanizing language he uses to describe nonautonomous persons belies that sentiment. He is not referring specifically to children in these examples (but to those with drug addictions, among others—should we be comforted?). But nowhere does he retract his damning portrait of nonautonomy.

Adams equates dignity with autonomy. The dignity of being autonomous is "*actual* dignity, based on qualities of character that will be actively manifested by whoever possesses autonomy."[21] He makes clear that this is very different from the imputed dignity wantonly distributed to all human beings, regardless of who actually deserves it. While he gives a nod to the moral advancements we have made by respecting everyone's imputed dignity, this is not real dignity in his eyes. Imputed dignity, as that which is given to a child because they are human, is not real dignity until the capacities underpinning that dignity have been brought to fruition. This has grave implications for the subjects of this book: Children with life-limiting illness, according to Adams, will never receive this actual dignity.

In this scheme, then, the true dignified moral subject is the one who achieves the goal of human flourishing: to be fully in control of one's own life. Being fully autonomous is essentially the same as being extremely privileged: One must have good genetics, all the benefits of a cosmopolitan upbringing, and no illness, tragedy, or accident to slow one down. And, crucially, being fully autonomous means *not being a child.* Compare this goal with the entangled and eschatological childhood described in the previous chapter, where the goal of human discipleship is to become like a child, and to live eternally as a child of God.

This deficiency view of childhood, as I think it is fair to characterize Adams's work, is reinforced in developmental psychology, which often sets the "scientific" benchmark for children's capabilities. Developmental psychology, like utilitarian and deontological moral theories, is a "paradigmatically *modern* discipline."[22] Children are viewed as amoral or proto-moral because morality requires abstract thought in order to determine the principles of action, according to medical ethics and other dominant theories. And we "know" from Jean Piaget, a twentieth-century founding father of modern childhood psychology, children are incapable of abstract thought. This is in some ways, of course, an oversimplification. For one thing, Piaget's importance is largely downplayed in contemporary developmental psychology, and his conclusions have been challenged. But Piaget "remains the dominant psychological resource for professionals who want to know 'how children think.'"[23]

For me, story makes it easier to grasp the distinction between these two competing ways of thinking, childist ethical intentionality versus autonomous subjectivity. George MacDonald's *Phantastes*, a sweeping and sometimes disorienting novel that can read like several short vignettes strung together, is an immersive experience in the myopia of narrow rationalism. Heavily influenced by Novalis and German Romanticism, the novel follows a young man named Anodos who is fresh from his "completed" education—and thrown into fairyland to learn properly. Anodos journeys from narrow-mindedness to a proper vision of reality, a reality that necessarily includes the feminine and the childlike. Eschewing cohesion and rational connections, MacDonald's novel is in line with the Romantic rejection of, and challenge to, the Enlightenment project, which prized the cold male intellect. What Anodos (and hopefully the reader) must cultivate are skills naturally possessed by children—namely, imagination, proper affective response, and a flexibility of thought that can comprehend the miraculous. Like critics of autonomy, MacDonald depicts Anodos, who has accepted a narrow, rationalist view of the world, as incapable of seeing reality in its entirety and thus of recognizing the good or trusting those who are worthy of trust.

But challenging an individualist and overly rationalist approach is not in and of itself sufficient to correct our preconceptions about children. Recent explorations in child ethics and theology of children helpfully challenge this autonomous moral vision, but in doing so they have at times eclipsed the moral subject and agent entirely. These thinkers have largely considered a child's ability to exercise a particular capacity, such as creativity or vulnerability, and disregarded her ability to appropriate herself as one who seeks and does the good in an integrated way. I take as my example of this larger trend John Wall, to whom I am indebted for the term "childist" as well as countless insights.[24] Despite the strengths of his project in *Ethics in the Light of Childhood*, it fails to adequately reimagine the moral subject, and thus to fundamentally transform ideas of moral agency so that children can be seen as genuine moral subjects and agents.

There are several problems with Wall's project. One is that Wall simply replaces rational capacity with the capacity for creativity. He argues that children, if we observe them, act for themselves in the world. Since they lack reason, reason cannot sufficiently account for this, thus it must be creativity that properly defines human moral being. While Wall talks about the many ways we can observe children acting in moral ways in the world, he ties this agency not to action, or even to subjectivity, but to the creation of worlds of meaning. Setting aside the question of whether children are truly equally creative as adults—are we considering spontaneous new ideas or the sustained creativity of Picasso's *Guernica*?—this focus on creativity in the abstract leads to an abstracted moral goal.

For Wall, the goal of the moral life is to be open to others so that we can create ever more expansive worlds of meaning. Lacking a clear notion of the subject, Wall has no clear definition of "meaning," or what is signified by "worlds of meaning." What Wall does not make clear, and perhaps cannot make clear because his work is not grounded in subjectivity, is that meaning can only arise from subjects, and thus children's developing subjectivity must be taken into account.[25] In his work, worlds of meaning seem to take priority over meaning-makers, and the value of creativity is to create ever-expanding worlds of meaning rather than meaningful ethical selfhood that is shared and communicated with others.

This means that in Wall's work, there is no criteria beyond "expansiveness" for determining meaning, and so it is not clear how one can judge what narratives or actions are moral. For example, if expansiveness is the goal, how do we reject the ancient cultural narrative that sees the practice of pederasty as educational? It would, after all, greatly expand a child's experience. The "teacher's" too, perhaps. I am not suggesting for an instant that Wall would be in favor of this. He speaks out strongly against child abuse in the book. But what I am saying is that he has given no procedural or substantive tools to argue against it—other than the idea of "responsiveness to the other." But it is unclear in his account what amounts to appropriate responsiveness, and how we know what erases or destroys the other. Underlying Wall's rejection of child abuse is something very much like the harm principle.

Similarly, he defines "pure agency" as the lack of limitations and vulnerability, and so declares that neither children nor adults have it. This is a confusing move; there's nothing inherent to human agency that should suggest its lack of limitation, and by capitulating the term in this way, he perpetuates the notion that moral agency is predicated on the autonomous notions of individuality and limitlessness.[26] Thus, in actual instances of moral conflict, we are left with a principlist approach predicated on the autonomous subject as the model of agency.

Instead, I think that childhood observed and recollected shows that children act meaningfully in the world in moral ways, not as contributors to general worlds of meaning, but as embodied moral selves in relationship who appropriate their moral subjectivity through a developing ethical intentionality. Children are a potent reminder of just how deeply personal human beings are. We begin life not only in worlds of meaning, but in the very body and loving embrace of another. This does not discount moral meaning but situates meaning as arising in and communicated between persons. Children exude self-expansion in loving relationships, not in abstract creation of meaning. Openness to others is thus about loving relationship with others, rather than the creation of worlds of meaning. And in this double beginning I talked about in the previous chapter, they live the goal of human life, which is relationship with God, who is true goodness.

In contrast to an ethics predicated on the autonomous subject who is moral primarily through the creation of principles and rules, and in contrast to an ethics that prizes expanding moral worlds of meaning, the child as moral subject reveals a deeply personal and shared ethics, where moral selfhood is appropriated and developed. This understanding of ethics must be understood as grounded in our existence as creatures and children of God. It is personal because moral meaning and moral action is rooted in the subject who is herself constituted by others. That is, morality is not a set of principles or a set of ideas, but rather arises in each person in relation to each other and to goodness itself, God. Ethics does not happen in abstract worlds of meaning, but in the subjectivity of each child.

This is why understanding children as intersubjective subjects who share in the human structure of ethical intentionality is crucial to understanding them as genuine moral subjects and agents. In this way, I hope to unite the communication of meaning, the use of moral language, and theories of action and intention with the responsible moral subject who continues through time.[27] The subject who can know herself and narrate her story through time is the agent of action; this narration is not tied to autonomy, nor to abstract worlds of meaning, but comes to fruition in the individual who exists in loving community.

But where I differ from Lonergan and Byrne, though I believe it can be justified in their work, is that I claim that this pursuit of the good is an eschatological pursuit characterized by our childhood in God. Where Byrne sets the "ideal of ethical authenticity" in self-appropriation, "knowing and valuing what it is to be a knower, valuer, and chooser, and choosing to act in accordance with that valued structure of knowing, valuing, and choosing,"[28] I believe that what is more important is our self-appropriation as children of God. To prevent bias and decline both in ourselves, and in our shared communal insights, we must constantly return to childhood, to cultivate the goods and relationships that characterize this double beginning and eschatological goal.

This means that our ethical intentionality should be structured by the goods of childhood. Only in this way can all human beings live out the goal of life, which is our childhood in God. And only in this way can we understand children as genuine moral subjects and agents who not only receive the moral world and develop, but who have something to teach us and who are properly our companions in the shared pursuit of the good.

***

The child as intersubjective moral subject is a moral agent because *she acts*. This includes, but is not limited to, acts of meaning. Moral subjectivity and agency are deeply linked: Children become patterned by experience, understanding, reasoning, and judgment, into particular persons who act according to their formation, their spontaneous intersubjectivity, their interpersonal relationships, and their endless creativity. So, then, children are moral agents because they are already in relationship with God, who is good, with others to whom they respond in ethical ways. Children are moral agents because they choose to seek and act according to the good through the operations of their ethical intentionality. By *attending to the moral agency of children in light of the goods of childhood*, we are reminded of the richness and variety of moral sources, types of reasoning, and moral language. In fact, to properly know and do the good, adults need to learn to be like children. Insofar as this structure is creative, affective, and imaginative, children bring specific strengths to ethical intentionality.

Furthermore, we know that children are moral agents because we can observe and witness this: they can do the right thing for the right reason. They respond affectively to others and work to act rightly. Take, for example, Gareth Matthew's story of Michael, aged fifteen months, and Paul:

> [Michael] was struggling with his friend, Paul, over a toy. Paul started to cry. Michael appeared concerned and let go of the toy so that Paul would have it, but Paul kept crying. Michael paused, then gave his teddy bear to Paul, but the crying continued. Michael paused again, then ran into the next room, returned with Paul's security blanket, and offered it to Paul, who then stopped crying.[29]

What has happened here? First, Michael is fighting with his friend. Children are not innocent or idealized moral actors but flawed human beings. They too can be selfish, petty, and mean, or simply thoughtless. Paul begins crying and Michael, observing this, seeks a response. He has an insight—that giving the toy to Paul will stop him from crying—and tests this insight, which fails. He then reasons that his teddy helps him feel better and gives it to Paul. No success. He then recalls that Paul has a security blanket and has another insight: that Paul's blanket is analogous to his teddy, and thus giving Paul his blanket may help. This insight he tests also, and it is successful.[30] Michael's reasoning leads him to judgment, and to decide on a course of action.

Not only that, but there is no adult ordering Michael to help Paul stop crying, nor is Michael acting on some abstract principle or duty. This is an internal response of Michael's, an affective response that leads to ethical action. Michael's affective response is not just the motivation added onto his ethical reflection and action. He does not first think of what can and should be done, and then dig around for the motivation to do it. Instead, his affective response to Paul's sadness underpins and sustains his entire series of actions, and even shapes his deliberation, in that he values a comfort for Paul akin to the comfort he receives from his special object.

Michael did not appear from nowhere as an ethical agent in this story. His ethical intentionality demonstrates his openness to moral sources other than rationality, sources like imitation and the development of moral language. This is part of what I meant earlier when I talked about the reception of morality. Michael may have seen adults doing the same things he is now doing to stop a fight and to comfort a crying child. He is creatively imitating an action he has likely received many times: that of a parent comforting him with his teddy bear. Imitation is a key aspect of ethics and plays a role in both communicating moral meaning and patterning our experiences and affective response. Children watch and imitate our moral actions long before they are aware of them as moral actions, or as being actions undertaken for specific reasons. If we start from an understanding of humans as intersubjective beings, we can see imitation as resulting from our beginning as nurtured inside the body of another, born into an existing matrix of moral aims and obligations, already having spontaneous affective response to others.

As a child, Michael is a powerful observer and imitator. One of the reasons that children are formed ethically by habituation is that they already spontaneously imitate and spontaneously react to other human beings. They are recipients of communicative acts of meaning.[31] This readiness to imitate, almost unconsciously held by children, shapes their experience, and allows them to appropriate the reasonings, actions, moral terminology, and judgments of others. To put this in Matthews's language, through imitation, children receive and expand their paradigms, range of cases, adjudication of conflict, and their moral imagination. This imitation is not the result of blindly following another, as it were, but can be understood in terms of our subjectivity: Children experience and observe the actions of others, they experience how they feel when those actions are directed toward them, they formulate ideas about what people around them are doing, and they understand themselves to be obligated to act in this way.

Think of how a toddler learns to be "gentle" with a new baby. We repeat the word over and over, a word which may at first have no meaning to them (to the disadvantage of our nostrils and glasses). This repetition is paired with actions: We touch the baby in a gentle way. Maybe we touch the toddler in the same way, so that they can feel it, and perhaps we touch them also in a non-gentle way, so that they learn the opposite. We encourage them to make the same sort of gentle movements we make. When toddlers learn to be gentle, they first learn the motions demonstrated to them. They do not stop there, however. They will begin to invent and try out their own gentle actions, like carefully laying a hankie over the baby's head, or stroking them with a wooden block. They may even admonish their parents and others for not being gentle enough with the baby.

This imitation is not limited to moral action but includes moral language as well. In the same way that children have an innate capacity for language, they have an innate capacity to "learn the inwardness of all sorts of ways of going on."[32] In their moral environment, which includes all that speaks to a child and to which the child reacts with intelligence and feeling, children not only receive moral training but engage with moral language and description. As Elizabeth Anscombe explains: "To grow up as a child of normal intelligence in a human society is *eo ipso* to be equipped with a range of concepts which form the raw material for moral action descriptions, and in many cases to acquire these as well at least in a rough inchoate form."[33] All humans grow up with a host of descriptions (lying, murder, generosity) which are already moral descriptions, which in turn shape their experiences, understandings, reasonings, judgments, and actions.

Moral action is tied to moral language; language is a key element in mediating our experience, understanding, and arrival at a judgment about a course of action. Children engage creatively with language, moral language included, and help adults to creatively reevaluate language. They often do this through play. Matthews notes how often children engage in *asteismus*, the intentional (comedic) misinterpretation of words.[34] Think back to the example about children and lying: Children will play with the notion of a lie by playing with the term, through the naming of opposites, and through nonsense terms. One notable area where we can see this occur is in the fantastical: Fantasy provokes the imagination through playing with the boundaries of language. Children, especially young children, regularly flit between fact and fantasy, making them ideal models for this kind of linguistic play.[35]

Against adult rigidity, MacDonald in his fairy tales encourages a child-likeness that can hold together a plurality of meaning, as described by U.C. Knoepflmacher:

> Instead of demanding hierarchies of meaning, children not only are willing to entertain multiple perspectives, but actually find great delight in the yoking of irreconcilables. They are therefore attracted to puns and homonyms, and to the instability of representations of the porous "borders" which MacDonald uses as a setting for so many of his fairy tales—narratives that are at once serious and playful, grave and light. MacDonald therefore invites his adult readers to adopt the same elasticity and open-mindedness that come so naturally to the child.[36]

Being literal-minded is, for MacDonald, an adult limitation, as embodied by Adela Cathcart's aunt in the book whose title bears her name. In the story,

Adela's uncle must use fairy tales to rescue the twenty-one-year-old protagonist "from giving in to a death-wish caused by her inability to find meaning or emotional sustenance in the denuded world around her."[37] Fairy tales help us to abandon the limited constructions of reality, including the moral reality, we have inherited. They mean more than meets the ear.

Thus, fairy tales act as places for adults and children to encounter and appropriate this fantastical approach. They also serve as imaginative vehicles for depicting the specific strengths children bring to the moral life. One of my favorite examples of this occurs in MacDonald's *The Princess and the Goblin*.[38] The mountain on which Princess Irene's palace is built, and in which the boy Curdie mines, is full of goblins who hold a grudge against the king. The goblins are planning an invasion of the king's house in order to kidnap Irene as a bride for their horrid prince Harelip. Curdie, who rescues Irene and her nurse one night on the mountainside, observes the unusual behavior of the goblins and bravely sneaks into their caves in the mountains to discover their plan. In this story, Irene and Curdie find themselves facing perils not of their own making, but respond bravely nonetheless. They exhibit creativity, resilience, and the ability to make life-changing decisions.

They exhibit this creativity and moral agency in specifically childlike ways. Curdie is not afraid of the goblins because he knows they fear happy nonsense and silliness. He invents creative ditties to repel them, and his nonsense is central to his fearlessness. Both Irene and Curdie explore and observe their surroundings and, without the expectations of adults, see things the adults around them miss. Irene and Curdie exhibit the strengths of childhood also in their reliance on the help of others. Irene is able to rescue Curdie from the mountain because she listens to her great-grandmother and has faith that enables her to follow the invisible string. Curdie receives wise teaching and guidance from his parents. They do not hold him back from his mission to find out what the goblins are scheming, but neither do they leave him to face the danger alone. Importantly, and this is often lost in reflections on children because we tend to see children through the paradigm of the adult-child relationship, Irene and Curdie work together to accomplish their goal. They strengthen, comfort, and admonish each other. They are even willing to sacrifice for each other.

The fantastical provides an example of how children, in their capacity for creative meaning-making and imagination, invite a reconsideration of the moral life. Fairy tales make this obvious, but if we attend to the children in our own lives, we can see the same invitation. Imagination is not antithetical to moral reasoning, but rather part of it. It is imagination that allows us to hold a plurality of meanings, to find new ways to envision moral situations and possibilities, and to find new ways of coming to judgment. As Wall puts it, "Children are simply the newest in the world, and so can play in the world in relatively more creative ways. They may not so easily take comfort in metaphysical or literal explanations or, on the contrary, world-denying cynicism."[39] I will return to the importance of the fantastical and the multiplicity of meaning in the next chapter on child death.

This flexibility expands beyond moral language to moral thinking more generally. All people become more patterned in their ways of thinking over time. This can be an advantage, as with the ornithologist who can almost instantly identify a bird, thanks to repeated patterns of understanding and judging. But it can also lead to stagnation, to seeing things as they have always been seen. If reaching judgment requires us to ask and answer relevant questions, when we refuse to see or entertain new questions, we risk coming to the wrong judgment. Children bring new vision.[40] Children ask new questions and challenge assumptions.[41] And they are surprisingly insightful about well-reasoned excuses.

Children are moral agents because they act in moral ways. But it can be easy to miss this in the busyness of life because our vision is patterned by our expectations. In the same way that we are accustomed to thinking about moral subjectivity in terms of the autonomous subject, we are used to considering the moral agent as the *autonomous agent*. The autonomous agent is one who acts according to his reason. He first deliberates. This deliberation is abstract, objective, and stripped of emotion. In some theories, the autonomous agent acts according to duty or principle against his own desires. This agent can offer systematic explanations for the reasoning behind his actions. This agent sets aside bias toward his family or his own relationships and seeks to treat everyone as equal.

Once again, it is not this book's project to offer a careful analysis of the nuances within moral theories of autonomy, nor to deal with the many challenges to this view. What is pertinent here is to see how, in this view, children cannot be genuine moral agents. Children lack the rational capacities required (by someone like Kant) to legislate the moral law for themselves according to the categorical imperative. Children do not treat others as equal, thus failing to be the objective observer of utilitarian theories. Instead, they are concerned with their own family and friends. At the same time, they often offer spontaneous generous acts of love to complete strangers, seemingly at random. Children respond emotionally. When they act, it is not clear that they have deliberated, nor can they explain their actions in systematic ways. They cannot reason abstractly about concepts they have never encountered.

While autonomy as a goal of human flourishing is, I think, completely incompatible with the childist account of moral subjectivity and agency I have been describing in this chapter, I do not mean to reject any notion of autonomy in terms of responsible moral action and self-appropriation as moral agent. That is, autonomy as a goal of moral selfhood is a problem, but there is an important way in which a limited autonomy is necessary to agency. A child wills from their own will. You can lead children to water, water they asked for just two minutes ago in the orange cup and everything, but you cannot make them drink. They are in part responsible for their own formation, though in a qualified sense. Children are not a product determined by their biological and social heritage. They can and should be actively involved in the construction of their own lives—a mediating process, if an asymmetrical one, that enriches parents and children who learn from each other by nature of their interdependence.

This autonomy is limited because of our double beginning: We begin life in relationship to other people, from whom we receive morality, and to God, the ultimate source of moral law. To will the good, for humans, is always to align our will with God's, not as an abdication of our freedom but as a realization of its proper end. While we do not determine what is the good, we play an active and creative role in working out that good in the world.[42] This role is not undertaken by isolated individuals, but by communities. It is in these communities that we inherit moral language, values, and obligations—they are an entire moral horizon into which we are born and that we hold even before we become aware of it. But a proper childlike autonomy sees that we interdependent humans have a partially autonomous role to play in our own moral lives and the working out of God's laws.

As I argued in the previous chapter, childhood is not only a double beginning, but also the eschatological goal of the Christian life. Childhood is not left behind after a certain period of time but persists throughout our lives. In order to love God, we must learn to be the children of God. As we age, we gain skills, experience, and abilities. But we also are at risk of losing our childlikeness in God as we seek to "shape and govern everything on [our] own."[43] As we grow in our self-appropriation as ethical agents, we also risk becoming patterned in wrong ways. We can become beholden to wrong understandings and judgments which then bias our experiences and perception of the world. We make the mistake of thinking that the way things are is the way things ought to be. Most of all, as we grow in our own abilities, we run the risk of believing that we legislate the moral law for ourselves, that we have control over ourselves, others, and the world.

Thus, a personal account of moral agency, grounded as it is in who we are as human beings, would be incomplete without a discussion of love. The radical dependency of love for God and others must be the goal of ethical intentionality. We don't make the moral law for ourselves, but we creatively engage with what God has revealed about the good. For Lonergan, "love transforms the way we experience the world. When we fall in love, we not only have new commitments, new judgments, and new ideas, but also new ways of being sensitive and spontaneously intersubjective."[44] Love, like the love between parents and children, transforms the ways that we experience the world and opens up new acts of meaning. Childhood lived, observed, and recollected reveals children as moral agents and subjects, and reveals the importance of the childlike, loving and dependent as it is, in the structure and goal of ethical intentionality.

***

Children are moral subjects and agents who share in the same structure of ethical intentionality as people of all other ages. Moreover, by attending to the goods of childhood in the moral life, we can see that there are particular strengths children bring to moral inquiry.

This means that children are properly our partners in moral deliberation and in seeking the good. But it is equally improper and dangerous to treat children in the same way we might treat other adults, especially if our idea of a full, responsible person is characterized by a narrow view of rational deliberation and objective judgment. Children contribute to shared moral inquiry in part because they are different. Older people, including older children and adolescents (though to a lesser extent), are obligated to nurture the ethical intentionality of children. This means properly guiding children in what is right, providing them with moral examples to imitate, paying attention to their experiences and insights, engaging them in dialogue, not lying to them, and not belittling their abilities.

The parent-child relationship, and by extension all adult-child relationships, is asymmetrical. This is true even of many child-child relationships. These relationships are how children receive the moral world, even as they challenge and reshape it. It is thus crucial that we pass on what is right, and that we encourage their formation in a proper way. The evidence that babies prefer helpers to hinderers, discussed above, has led some researchers to suggest that a natural biological orientation of right and wrong resides in each person.[45] But even if this is true, it does not exist in isolation from the relationships, concepts, examples, and moral language that a child receives. Michael is able, in part, to respond to Paul because he has paradigms for comfort and for helping. Irene and Curdie are able to be brave because they are supported by the people around them. Irene's great-grandmother teaches Irene and inspires her with the desire to be good. Similarly, Curdie's parents respect and nurture his abilities, provide support, and guide him.

Despite the goods of childhood that they bring to moral inquiry, children are also dependent on adults for their moral formation, and are limited in their cognitive, emotional, physical, and spiritual development. Because of the asymmetry of the adult-child relationship, when we talk about shared meaning between children and adults, we have to recognize that these acts of meaning will often be different. When children communicate meaning and adults respond, the adults may be responding on a different level than that communicated. For example, children may communicate on the level of experience in inchoate ways and adults will respond on the level of reason or judgment. Thus, we must recognize that to expect some levels of moral reasoning or some types of decisions from children—independent of guidance—will harm them, because it asks more from them then they are capable of giving.

Further, children are vulnerable to the models of imitation they receive and the language taught to them. In the same way that children can learn virtue by imitation and habituation, so too can they learn vice. Often, they learn it through mistaken moral description. Anscombe discusses the importance of proper discretion and description in situations involving children. She gives the example of stealing: Many young children steal, and this should be treated not by stringent methods but by restitution. Most importantly, it is important not to "call theft anything that is mere disobedience and greed within a family."[46] It is inappropriate to hold children to moral absolutes that do not take into account descriptions of actions given to a child, or that assume adult motivations for childish acts. In stories, we see this too. Not all adults are so helpful: Curdie tries to warn the guards about the goblin invasion but is ignored and imprisoned instead. Irene's nurse is similarly unwilling to listen to the princess and calls Irene's goodness disobedience.

Children are similarly vulnerable because they are so often excluded from opportunities to develop reason and to receive correction; because reasoning becomes patterned over time, exclusion can cause them to become habituated in poor reasoning.[47] Understanding children as moral agents who share in our moral world does not mean that we simply see them as miniature adults; instead, we have a responsibility to guide, nurture, and protect children while remaining open to what they have to teach us. Children do not think just like adults, even if they share in the same structures of conscious and ethical intentionality. I think it is important to recognize that their thinking is qualitatively different to some extent, though not completely different, as imagined in many stage theories. There are obvious differences between children and adults, as the goods of childhood demonstrate.

A child's ability to grow in the knowledge of and the desire for the good is significantly affected by their environment. Because the moral world is first received from others, and then creatively responded to, the reasonings, judgments, language, and examples children receive play a significant role in shaping their moral being. So too does the effort we put into training them in the operations of ethical intentionality. In her anthropology of childhood, Heather Montgomery describes how our expectations of children often determine our assessment of their capabilities. She explains that North American society today considers it impressive if a child of four years of age can tie her own shoes. But a few hundred years ago, it was normal for a child of that age to be embroidering and knitting items for the household. The difference between children then and now is not their innate developmental capacities, but the time that others take to teach them such skills.[48]

Similarly, children's moral abilities are shaped by the effort we put into their development and the time we spend nurturing the operations of their ethical intentionality, far more than by the limitations of their innate capacities, as stage theories depict. The difference between these two ways of thinking can be seen in the approaches of Piaget and Lev Vygotsky. Instead of seeing development, as Piaget did, as preceding learning—that is, development of capacities for knowledge as the "unfolding of some genetic or neurological imperative"—Vygotsky described the acquisition of knowledge capacity as a primarily social endeavor.[49] Learning is foundational to development.

This learning unfolds through social collaboration, through the dialogical process between the child and others, whether more advanced peers or adults. Children can achieve much more in collaboration with others than they can if left to their own devices.

To put this another way, there is a difference between respect and disinterest. Consider the Norwegian educational reform of the 1990s, in which the new pedagogical model required students, especially older ones, to be responsible for their own education.[50] I have no problem with this in theory. But the questions that should immediately spring to mind are: *Where and how did they learn what it means to be responsible for one's own education? Were they trained in it, given a chance to explore paradigms of responsibility, to consider different cases? Are they allowed to exercise this responsibility in other aspects of their lives, or are we compartmentalizing their development?* Learning to take responsibility is a skill that requires development. And it is one thing to expect students to take initiative; it is another entirely to expect them to know how to learn, as if scholarly skills of research, reading, writing, grammar, and clear argumentation reside innate inside every child waiting for release.

Respecting children as genuine moral agents does not mean that we need to say, as Wall does, that children can act for themselves just as well as adults.[51] In the spirit of Aristotle on virtue and skill, we can think of moral development as comparable to learning household chores. Consider a common model for teaching children to do chores: First, they watch you complete the task (often when it sparks their interest and desire); second, they do it with you; third, they do it on their own with supervision; finally, they do it on their own. Biological development does not in itself give a child the know-how to properly use a broom, nor does it teach them the difference between types of brooms and in which direction they should push them to clean effectively. In the same way, even if children from infancy display a preference for moral good, as the babies who prefer helpers do, this inclination does not by itself give them the tools of moral discernment. As with proper sweeping technique, they may in time figure it out for themselves. But while seeing someone ineffectively sweep dirt toward themselves with a push broom is mildly amusing, the stakes in moral development are significantly higher.

The example of sweeping is pertinent in another way. The biggest limitation to a child's ability to sweep a floor is not her lack of coordination. It is the fact that most household brooms are sized for adults. Give a three-year-old a small broom, and she does much better. In like manner, when we engage in moral deliberation with children, we should consider whether our approach fits their needs. Michael could not have described his moral actions in the way I have in this chapter. He likely has no idea that there is a concept we call morality to which his actions conform. If he has a concept of the good, he certainly cannot express it in the form of literal statement or philosophical treatise. But this does not mean we cannot communicate effectively with him about morality. Parents, researchers, teachers, and siblings use a whole variety of means to communicate with children, including bodily movements (that allow children to play out their feelings and desires), arts and crafts, stories, nearness, and so on.

Because children share in the same structure of ethical intentionality that we do, and because childhood is not a discrete stage but continues through our lives, this moral education should be mutual, if asymmetrical. Children can and do act in ways that defy their situations, like Naaman's little servant girl. Instead of venerating adulthood as the pinnacle of full, responsible ethical agency, we must remember that moral development continues through our lives, beginning in our first childhood and aiming toward childhood in God. Guiding children does not require us to be ideal actors either, because we too can be challenged and converted. This is not Adams's vision of flourishing as wealthy, cosmopolitan, unencumbered people. Rather, we learn to be in relationship with true goodness through crises and difficulties as well, because loving relationship is the goal of the moral life, not control.

Most importantly, properly nurturing children's moral development means setting aside our tendency to belittle and underestimate their abilities. Instead, we ought to recognize their genuine contributions. In this way, we can see them as our partners in the shared task of knowing and loving the good. Think of the delight on the face of some babies or young children every time someone looks at them. As I write this, my younger daughter is nine months old. Every time someone looks at her, her whole face lights up. She flails her arms and legs and rocks back and forth as her whole body communicates her utter joy in seeing the face of another. I could dismiss this response as a predictable stage in her development or be anxious that she is not hitting the developmental milestone where this reaction becomes limited to people that she knows. Or I could cynically observe how exhausting it looks to be so stoked all the time (no wonder she takes two naps a day!).

But if I take this as a genuine affective and moral response to others, I should ask myself: *What if her response is the proper response to the face of*

*another? Is she immature, or have I allowed myself to become numb to the abso-
lute miracle of every human being who is made in God's image?* Her reaction
has made me rethink what Levinas said about the moral demand inherent
to the face-to-face encounter with the other. I have always thought of this
grimly, as a necessity in light of deep human cruelty. But the delight on my
daughter's face has invited me to reflect that the moral exigence in the face
of the other can be experienced not as a demand but as a joyful response, an
ecstatic indulgence in the wonder that is another person.

In this way, we can see the things that we lose, or are in danger of losing,
when we become adults. Anscombe begins her essay on transubstantiation by
saying that it can be summed up in the statement "little children should be
taught about it as early as possible."[52] We teach this concept to a young child,
not by using fancy terms, but by explaining the conversion of one physical
reality into another: bread into Jesus. Against the adult tendency to overin-
tellectualize (and then lose their faith in the event), children grasp both the
concept and the act of worship that follows: "I knew a child, close upon three
years old and only then beginning to talk, but taught as I have described,
who was in the free space at the back of the church when the mother went to
communion. 'Is he in you?' the child asked when the mother came back. 'Yes,'
she said, and to her amazement the child prostrated itself before her."[53] What
a rebuke to those of us who eat the bread week after week, barely discerning
the body of Christ, let alone worshipping it as is deserved.

This does not mean that my child (or the child in Anscombe's story) is
some sort of philosophical and theological genius who can reveal all the
truths of human life. Nor does it mean that she does not also pull hair or fight
over toys. But she is not simply an object of my own moral reflection, either.
Instead, we have participated in a genuine encounter of shared meaning,
where her spontaneous reaction has woken my own moral imagination to
consider anew both the writings of a particular author and, more generally,
what it means to love others. As Matthews puts it, "A child's naïve question
can awaken our sleeping imagination and sympathy, and even move us to
take moral action."[54]

Children wake us through their endless observation, explorations, and
"why" questions. Studies show that four-year-olds ask two hundred to three
hundred questions a day.[55] Similarly, they demonstrate a keen interest in
responding to the emotions, feelings, and needs of others. They also wake us
through their imitation. Sometimes they simply embody the moral actions

of their parents, as when they imitate physical calming motions. This is not mere mimicry, but rather sharing in the intention in the action—that is, children exhibit a desire to act in these ways. But this mimicry can also be morally informative for those around them. I recall a friend telling the story of his young sister commenting, after their family car had been cut off by a female driver, "Somebody needs to get laid." It was mortifying for his parents, who were suddenly made aware of how they spoke about other drivers. Our gestures, habits, and common phrases are all reflected back to us in the behavior of our children, in amusing ways, but also in morally serious ways. This imitation confronts us with who we are and what we are passing on to others.

Because children and adults share in the same structure of ethical intentionality, and because we can communicate meaning to each other, and because infants, children, adolescents, young adults, and the elderly all excel at different operations, we can think of moral deliberation and action as a shared endeavor. This vision does not discount the importance of individuals seeking the good and trying to act rightly for themselves. But it does mean that we can properly make decisions *together* in a way that does not diminish the agency of another. As Gareth Matthews found by doing philosophy with children, children raise questions and theories beyond the answers of the adults around them: "if [children] can raise for us in vivid and compelling form the puzzles of how the universe could have begun, then there are at least some contexts in which they should be considered our partners in a joint effort to understand it all."[56] Children, as moral subjects and agents who share in the same structure of ethical intentionality as all human beings and who model what it means to be children of God, are properly our partners in the shared human task of knowing and loving the good.

NOTES

1 Mark T. Miller, *The Quest for God and the Good Life: Lonergan's Theological Anthropology* (Washington DC: Catholic University of America Press, 2013), 39.

2 Marilyn Friedman, "Autonomy, Social Disruption, and Women," in *Relational Autonomy: Feminist Perspectives on Autonomy, Agency, and the Social Self,* ed. Catriona Mackenzie and Natalie Stoljar (New York: Oxford University Press, 2000), 35–51; Linda Barclay, "Autonomy and the Social Self," in *Relational Autonomy: Feminist Perspectives on Autonomy, Agency, and the Social Self,* ed. Catriona Mackenzie and Natalie Stoljar (New York: Oxford University Press, 2000), 54.

3 See, for example, Barclay, "Autonomy and the Social Self," 65–68.

4 Bernard Lonergan, *Method in Theology* (Toronto: University of Toronto Press, 1990), 9.

5 Lonergan, *Method*, 9.

6 Lonergan, *Method*, 133.

7 Miller, *Quest*, 73.

8 Patrick H. Byrne, *The Ethics of Discernment: Lonergan's Foundations for Ethics* (Toronto: University of Toronto Press, 2016), 95–96.

9 Byrne, *Ethics of Discernment*, 97.

10 Paul Bloom, *Just Babies: The Origins of Good and Evil* (New York: Random House, 2013), 50–56.

11 Byrne, *Ethics of Discernment*, 100.

12 Brock Bahler, *Childlike Peace in Merleau-Ponty and Levinas: Intersubjectivity as Dialectical Spiral* (New York: Lexington Books, 2016), 3–10.

13 Lonergan, *Method*, 76–77.

14 2 Kings 5. See Esther M. Menn, "Child Characters in Biblical Narratives: The Young David (1 Samuel 16–17) and the Little Israelite Girl (2 Kings 5:1–19)," in *The Child in the Bible*, ed. Marcia J. Bunge (Grand Rapids: Eerdmans, 2008), 343.

15 Cathleen Kaveny, *Law's Virtues: Fostering Autonomy and Solidarity in American Society* (Washington, DC: Georgetown University Press, 2012), 23–24.

16 See also Iris Murdoch, *The Sovereignty of Good* (New York: Routledge Classics, 2001), 78.

17 Cf. Lorraine Code, "The Perversion of Autonomy and the Subjection of Women: Discourses of Social Advocacy at Century's End," in *Relational Autonomy: Feminist Perspectives on Autonomy, Agency, and the Social Self*, ed. Catriona Mackenzie and Natalie Stoljar (New York: Oxford University Press, 2000), 182.

18 Harry Adams, *Justice for Children: Autonomy Development and the State* (Albany: State University of New York Press, 2007), 17–18.

19 Adams, 24.

20 Adams, 22.

21 Adams, 25, emphasis his.

22 Erica Burman, *Deconstructing Developmental Psychology*, 3rd ed. (London: Routledge, 2017), 243.

23 Burman, *Deconstructing Developmental Psychology*, 237.

24 John Wall, *Ethics in the Light of Childhood* (Washington, DC: Georgetown University Press, 2010).

25 Wall, *Ethics*, 59–86.

26 Wall, *Ethics*, 40–41.

27 Cf. Paul Ricoeur's critique of Anscombe. Paul Ricoeur, *Oneself as Another*, trans. Kathleen Blamey (Chicago: University of Chicago Press, 1992), 67–73.

28 Byrne, *Ethics of Discernment*, 297.

29 Gareth B. Matthews, *The Philosophy of Childhood* (Cambridge: Harvard University Press, 1994), 57.

30 Of course, I'm not suggesting that Michael would objectify his actions and be able to explain the sequence of events in this way. But the ability to use these operations is not reliant on the ability to objectify and study the operations themselves.

31 G. E. M. Anscombe, "The Moral Environment of a Child," in *Faith in a Hard Ground: Essays on Religion, Philosophy and Ethics by G. E. M. Anscombe*, ed. Mary Geach and Luke Gormally (Exeter: Imprint Academic, 2008), 229–230.

32 Anscombe, "Moral Environment," 224.

33 Anscombe, "Moral Environment," 225.

34 Gareth B. Matthews, *Philosophy and the Young Child* (Cambridge: Harvard University Press, 1980), 14.

35 V. Kudryavtsev, "The Imagination of the Preschool Child: The Experience of Logical-Psychological Analysis." *Journal of Russian & East European Psychology* 54 (2017): 393–401.

36 U. C. Knoepflmacher, "Introduction," in *The Complete Fairy Tales*, ed. U. C. Knoepfulmacher (New York: Penguin Books, 1999), x.

37 Knoepflmacher, "Introduction," xiii.

38 George MacDonald, *The Princess and the Goblin* (London: Puffin Classics, 2010).

39 Wall, *Ethics*, 54.

40 Wall, *Ethics*, 41; see also Bahler, *Childlike Peace*, 3–10.

41 Matthews, *The Philosophy of Childhood*, 65.

42 See Catriona Mackenzie and Natalie Stoljar, eds., *Relational Autonomy: Feminist Perspectives on Autonomy, Agency, and the Social Self* (New York: Oxford University Press, 2000). See also, for example, Thomas Reynolds, *Vulnerable Communion: A Theology of Disability and Hospitality* (Grand Rapids: Brazos Press, 2008), 180.

43 Hans Urs von Balthasar, *Unless You Become Like This Child*, trans. Erasmo Leiva-Merikakis (San Francisco: Ignatius Press, 1991), 43.

44 Miller, *Quest*, 79.

45 Bloom, *Just Babies*, 7–32.

46 Anscombe, "Moral Environment," 233.

47 Even here there is hope: Anscombe writes that even if it is a bad moral environment, "it will be full of matter which provides the raw material for the ethical." Anscombe, "Moral Environment," 233.

48 Heather Montgomery, *An Introduction to Childhood: Anthropological Perspectives on Children's Lives* (Chichester: Wiley-Blackwell, 2009), 56.

49 Michael K. White, *Maps of Narrative Practice* (New York: Norton, 2007), 271.

50 Val D. Rust, "The Policy Formation Process and Educational Reform in Norway" in *Comparative Education* 26 (1990): 13–25.

51 Wall, *Ethics*, 82.

52 G. E. M. Anscombe, "On Transubstantiation," in *Faith in a Hard Ground: Essays on Religion, Philosophy and Ethics by G. E. M. Anscombe*, eds. Mary Geach and Luke Gormally (Exeter: Imprint Academic, 2008), 84–86.

53 Anscombe, "On Transubstantiation," 84–86.

54 Matthews, *Philosophy of Childhood*, 65.

55 Telegraph Staff and Agencies, "Mothers asked nearly 300 questions a day, study finds," in *The Telegraph*, March 28, 2013. https://tinyurl.com/4evpwevu

56 Matthews, *The Philosophy of Childhood*, 13.

CHAPTER 3

Can a Child Die a Good Death?

Childhood seems antithetical to death. The unfolding of biological potential, the growth and expansion of cognitive ability, the very regular passage of time in which a child grows from a cluster of cells to a baby, then a toddler, and finally out of childhood into adolescence and adulthood all suggest that childhood is one stage of an ongoing human life. Children grow, mature, develop. Children, in their freshness and youth, seem to illustrate renewed hope and the future orientation of human life. Child death thus feels like a disruption of the natural course of events. As childhood mortality rates (thankfully) decrease, this sense of antithesis becomes even stronger.

In fact, child death challenges the very role of the child in Western culture. Here, the "protected child" dominates images of childhood. It is almost a self-justifying principle that parents ought to shield their children from knowledge of politics, war, sex, and death, on the basis that even knowing about these things causes suffering. Nonideal childhoods (whether the children who live them are impoverished, go to work, are caregivers, are in a war zone, or become sick) are deemed lost or thwarted.[1] Significantly, protection (from harm, exploitation, abuse) makes up the basis of the United Nations Convention on the Rights of the Child; officials only added participation rights (that is, the rights for children to make their views known) in the 1989 declaration.[2] This primacy of protection still holds sway in Western culture, and is increasingly normative in international policy. Yet as I mentioned in the first chapter, this view of children is both recent and narrow, arising out of particular cultural circumstances among privileged families in the eighteenth, nineteenth, and twentieth centuries. Nor has it gone unchallenged;

as one example, in the 1920s and 1930s, the BBC tailored its content to be clear enough for children to follow, with the idea that children were engaged listeners and active citizens.[3]

Child death also challenges the relational roles between children and adults, which are bound up with the goals of childhood. Children who are dying are experiencing a major life stage before their parents, and often their grandparents. Should not the parent go first, and model death to a child? In the face of death, the parental role of protecting and nurturing a child becomes impossible to fulfill. Similarly, child death thwarts the parental role of guidance: What we do with and for children is often oriented toward future goals, intended to help them become competent and contributing members of adult society.

In light of this antithetical relationship between childhood and death, the central question of this chapter might seem wrong. This chapter asks the question: *Can a child die a good death?* I have phrased it this way because the one question asks two different things: It asks what a given child with life-limiting illness experiences, and it asks what we perceive to be the "good death." These two considerations interlock in important ways. There are many moral and cultural ideals around death that prevent us from recognizing that children can die a good death. And what we communicate to children (implicitly or explicitly) about death and dying, and how children experience death itself, are intimately related.

To ask whether a child can die a good death is a different question from "is the death of a child good?" To this question I can give an emphatic answer. Death is never good, even in cases where children and their families are prepared for it and welcome it as the only alternative to living in pain and uncertainty. Death is not even good for those who believe that it has been transformed into a passageway to eternal life. George MacDonald, who wrote Diamond's story, held fast to this faith: "Oh dear, what a mere inn of a place the world is! and thank God! we must widen and widen our thoughts and hearts. A great good is coming to us all—too big for this world to hold."[4] And yet he still bitterly mourned the death of his three children.[5] Future hope does not prevent present grief.

Yet I argue that children can die a good death. They can do so because they are moral subjects and agents who make meaning and live in loving relationships with those around them. Most importantly, they already live the goal of Christian discipleship: They live as children of God. Children can die a good death when the good death is predicated on intersubjectivity, shared meaning-making, and presence. Hope for a good death is found not in control and conscious choice, but in who children (and who we all) are as human beings. Dying children and their caregivers can find hope in relationships, in honest speech, in attending to sources of suffering such as pain, in the endless possibilities for meaning-making present in our lives and deaths, and in lament. By openly and honestly communicating with children at the ends of their lives, we can hear their insights into their experiences, witness their creative moral responses, and reimagine together our new relational roles. We can comfort them, grieve with them, assuage their guilt, and reassure them that they are loved.

But in the face of the grief and suffering that accompanies the death and dying of children, the most common public reaction is avoidance. Dying children are sequestered away from public view in separate cultural spaces—that is, hospitals. The dominating medical and cultural image of a sick child is that of a fighter who triumphs over their illness, and the dominant narrative about the pediatric hospital system is a victorious story of cure, as in the ad campaign released by SickKids Toronto that I discussed in the introduction. This reaction fits into what Charles Taylor describes as a more general cultural trend: "We are much more sensitive to suffering, which we may of course just translate into not wanting to hear about it rather than into any concrete remedial action."[6]

Concrete remedial action begins by reconsidering the stories we tell about children, which I have challenged and to which I have offered alternatives in the first two chapters of this book, and by reconsidering the stories we tell about death. We have received a moral vision of death that is predicated on rational, autonomous choice. As I illustrated in the previous chapter, this narrow account of rationality, and the image of autonomy as rugged individualization, excludes all children. This is all the more true for children who are dying, and thus will never fulfill the vision of human personhood put forward by someone like Harry Adams. This vision underpins the medicalization of death, as the moral structures of the hospital reproduce this same focus on the rational, autonomous individual. Yet while children may not be rational, narrowly understood, nor autonomous, they can think about and understand death. Whether dying is a meaningful, transformative process, or whether dying is only given meaning by exercises of autonomous choice, greatly affects how we approach it. Our decisions in life are shaped by the stories we tell—this is no less true in death.

To create new stories around child death and address the concrete reality of a dying child, it is vital to attend to and communicate with children at the end of life. By "attend to" I mean listening, touching, playing with, and observing children, paying attention to all of the myriad communicative acts in which they engage, not only their words. When we understand children as fully human moral subjects and agents, we see clearly that the process of dying is not only medical but involves their whole personhood. Children have a range of feelings about themselves and their experiences of being ill. These feelings are real, intentional responses to values. They often have particular desires for what happens at their funeral, or how their worldly goods will be distributed. Listening to these desires, taking them seriously, and working alongside them is part of caring for dying children, as well as attending to their medical needs.

Attending to children also allows us to confront the nebulous notion of suffering that accompanies thought about children with life-limiting illness. Talking about suffering is not only difficult emotionally, but intellectually too, in part because suffering is recognizable as a category of experience, but it is not a *thing* or *type*. Suffering comes from many sources, causes, and experiences, and the relationship between cause and effect is not straightforward. We must tease these relationships out, to see how many sources of suffering can be confronted in the life of a dying child. Children with life-limiting illnesses in Western, industrialized countries encounter particular sources of suffering. In each of these cases, there are concrete steps that can be taken to confront the sources of suffering.

Unfortunately, this attending to children, and communicating openly and honestly with them, is frequently lacking in our medical institutions and our wider culture.[7] As I will explore in this chapter, this silence around death significantly affects the care that children receive, medically, emotionally, spiritually, and psychologically. The refusal to acknowledge that death is imminent and the inability to communicate with children result in increased suffering for sick children and their community. Few public rituals exist for recognizing and supporting dying children, their families, and their caregivers. Medical staff often report insufficient training in areas such as communicating about end-of-life issues and DNR discussions with families. In turn, families often identify callous communication by health-care professionals as a significant cause of distress.

We cannot expect children to die well in these circumstances. We cannot expect them to die well when we sequester them in protected spaces cut off from the rest of their society, as if their only needs at the end of life were confined to a hospital room. Nor can we expect them to participate well in their own care and dying without preparation and clear communication. We cannot assume that children will do well at something that they have no experience with. Thus, we have a responsibility to give them, according to their individual needs and situations, the tools to die well. Dying well is something done *together* with others (and God), and so we must both teach children and walk with them. But it is unfair to expect parents, grandparents, siblings, and other family members to overcome the dominant stories of their culture and be able to face honestly the death of their child. We cannot expect children's friends to offer support if the very notion of child death is frightening enough that their parents will prevent them from visiting.[8] And we cannot expect dedicated pediatric health-care workers to be able to meet the needs of dying children in such a world. For us to help children die well, we must transform medical culture and indeed the wider culture.

This chapter, then, is an invitation to reconsider what it means for a child to die a good death, and what they can teach us about what it means to die well. It is also a challenge for us to confront this issue in the wider culture, in our homes, churches, schools, and not just in the hospital. Ryan Green's video game *That Dragon, Cancer* invites players to follow Green's autobiographical experience of watching his son die of cancer. A *Wired* article about the game concludes: "He is making a game that is as broken—as confounding, unresolved, and tragically beautiful—as the world itself."[9] In one scene, players share Green's increasing desperation as every action taken to soothe his son fails. I do not pretend to offer any explanation for why this happens, to justify God's action. Such argument is outside my abilities. This chapter is not a theodicy. But I hope to do in a small way what this game does: to create cultural space for shared stories about child death, and to draw attention to stories and art forms that invite people to join in solidarity with the suffering of a parent.

This chapter will touch on issues around certain pediatric health-care practices, the state of research on child death, and children's access to palliative care. Mainly, though, I want to consider what it means for a child to die a good death in a culture that does not make space for dying children, because I believe that a hospital system that pursues cure at almost any cost is a product of a death-denying culture. I am hardly alone in this conviction; many articles on end-of-life care for children specifically reference the fact that child death is seen as unnatural.[10] That is, they link cultural notions of "naturalness" to the quality of care children receive. The insufficient training of medical staff is not simply an oversight in medical education, but an indicator of the state of medical care in a culture that hides child death and pretends it does not happen. The reality is that the hospital system, as amazing as it is, cannot provide the level of support needed by dying children, their families, and their medical caregivers.

Our hope for a good death, however, is never simply in the systems we devise. I end this chapter with a child-centered eschatology, which puts our hope ultimately not in medicine or even in human communities and support, as valuable as these are. Hope is found in a life made complete in God, and in the ways in which all human meaning, relationships, and love find their wholeness in Him. Children are already in relationship with God, in whom all stories find their completion and ultimate meaning. Remembering this is especially important when considering the dying child, whose truncated life can trigger grief over failed potential and lack of a meaningful life narrative. It is also from this child-centered eschatology, remembering that the goal of Christian discipleship is to be a child of God, that we acknowledge that *we should all die as children*. I don't want this misunderstood: I'm certainly not advocating for increased rates of child death! But in the same way that all children reveal something about what it means to be human, so too can dying children model for us what it means to die well.

So, then, by communicating openly with children at the end of life, we can help them befriend death by meeting their physical, emotional, and spiritual needs, and thus reducing as much as possible the painful symptoms of the dying process. We can help them befriend death too, by allowing them to use the dying process to bathe in loving relationship with their friends, families, and caregivers. And, together, we can learn how death can be befriended despite the pain and rupture it causes. Children, who are already in relationship with God, and already model discipleship, are powerful reminders that completion and hope are found in relationship with God who has promised to hold us in faithful love. Children teach us how to "welcome God, through Christ's call to welcome children."[11] This is no less true when they are dying.

∗∗∗

One of the remarkable things about the story *At the Back of the North Wind* is that it portrays the sustained dying of a child. As readers come to understand that North Wind is death, they understand that, in some ways, Diamond's first serious illness is the beginning of his dying process, even though he recovers from this illness and goes back to regular life for quite some time. In other ways, of course, this is not the case; we cannot identify the specific causal relationship between Diamond's initial sickness and his death. Diamond meets many other people who have encountered North Wind. Readers can presume that these people, too, suffered from a serious illness and are now recovered. Only time will tell whether that illness was the beginning of the dying process as well. This pattern will be familiar to children with illnesses that go through periods of remission.

For readers today, any portrayal of a child's death, especially a fictional portrayal of a child's relationship with the personification of death, is a rarity. Even among books written to help children understand grief, few talk specifically about child death. One website listing children's books about grief and death adds a special proviso about a book written by Michael Rosen about the death of his son, noting that it may be too advanced for young readers "who are not ready for discussions about the death of a child."[12] Perhaps we should ask who it is who is not ready for that discussion.

Even MacDonald's book does not portray, as Ryan Green's video game does, the concrete realities of Diamond's illness. MacDonald's book focuses on inspiring hope and possibility and tells us nothing of Diamond's experience of being sick in this world; we hear of his adventures with North Wind, not about his probable pain, fever, discomfort, or lack of appetite. This is because of the purpose of the book. As I explained in the introduction, MacDonald wrote this book in response to the changes in attitudes toward death in the Victorian period. The Victorian cult of death, with its photography of the dead, mausoleums, and grandiose mourning practices, had significant drawbacks of its own, stemming from a crisis of faith in the afterlife. As hope in the afterlife diminished, more and more focus was put on dying itself.[13] This preoccupation often had a strong moralizing character: Good boys and girls died peacefully, whereas bad ones died in agony. Dead children were arranged to look ethereal, angelic. Literary accounts of child deathbed scenes were replete at that time, but they did not go unchallenged. In *Jude the Obscure*, Thomas Hardy challenged the piety of the deathbed scene, and MacDonald, in *North Wind* and other writings, sought to reinforce belief in the afterlife. While we are in many ways far removed from the Victorian cult of death, this pristine and peaceful death is still the most common portrayal of child death on television today. This is one of the reasons I believe MacDonald's work still speaks to us: He was confronting similar cultural pressures around finding meaning in the dying and death of a child.

At the Back of the North Wind is also remarkable because it focuses on the child who is dying. While I make no comments here about the concrete circumstances of care for any given child, the medical and ethical literature on dying children often obscures the child who is at the center of it all. Children and their families are often treated as a unit, as though what is true of parents is also true of their children. Medical ethics tends to approach conflicts as matters between parents and physicians, or simply between competing moral principles. And because children have few participatory rights, their participation relies on the willingness of adults. Children take on a passive role in their illness and dying. In contrast, in MacDonald's story, Diamond is a moral subject and agent who is himself transformed through his encounters with North Wind. Like all children he is an intersubjective subject who can share meaning-making in his own familial and cultural milieu.

This meaning-making extends to their own death. It is well documented in pediatric literature that children communicate their own knowledge that they are sick and dying. They do so in words, using statements like "I know that I am dying" or "what is the point of this homework because I'm never going back to school."[14] They can use more oblique references, such as bringing up the children who had been in the same hospital ward and died previously. Children also communicate through nonverbal means. Some children draw pictures of funerals, of themselves in heaven or as angels, of graveyards and other objects associated with death. Some children bury their stuffed animals, treasured objects, siblings, or even themselves under the blankets of their beds. In these and other ways, children communicate with those around them the knowledge that they are going to die.

Children come to know about their illness and impending death whether or not they are directly informed about it. In Myra Bluebond-Langner's study, one child told her that he knew he was very ill rather than just sick the way children often are because his parents suddenly stopped disciplining him in the same way.[15] Children and adolescents also learn about the deaths of other children in their hospital ward through their own channels of communication. In the days of Bluebond-Langner's study, whispers between the children would spread the news that a child had died. In today's technological age, one mother recounted that she had tried to hide the death of another teen on the ward from her adolescent daughter. The daughter found out through Facebook and scolded her mother for hiding the news.[16]

Conversations about death are often initiated by children.[17] As intelligent beings with ethical and cognitive intentionality, they often seek to know about their condition and prognosis. In these encounters, children try to make meaning around death and dying. They do so in myriad ways: through conversation and art, reflecting on stories, fairy tales, memories of dead loved ones and pets, and ideas of heaven, as I will discuss in the following section. Some researchers report that "children often guide parents through the process of closure and saying goodbye."[18] Being present with children and attending to what they communicate allows us to explore together the meaning to be found in the dying process.

But despite the fact that children (try to) communicate about their impending deaths with their parents, many families and caregivers do not discuss death with their seriously ill child. This lack of discussion means that the child does not get to participate openly in the dying process with the support of their families, friends, and caregivers, and is often excluded from decision-making about their care. One reason for this is that families can be unable to acknowledge the medical reality of their child's illness. But even when families do recognize its seriousness, they cannot necessarily communicate any better with their child. Some of this difficulty can be attributed to the lack of supportive spaces, such as pediatric palliative care and hospices, and other cultural spaces for dying children and those who love them.[19]

This lack of engagement makes sense because we want to protect children from suffering. But the reality is that shielding children from knowledge of their death more often harms them—and harms their siblings and friends too. Franca Benini, Roberta Vecchi, and Marcello Orzalesi summarize the cost of such silence:

> But, it is the children who pay the highest price, suffering, and coping directly with the burden of incurable illness and death, the trauma of separation, the loss of their future, and often, in solitude, the consequences of their illness, fears, and emotions. Sometimes, the people closest to them refuse to accept the negative progression of the disease and, consequently, do not recognize terminal illness and death as real and imminent issues to be addressed. As a result, these children are subjected to unrealistic decisions and treatment choices. More

frequently, although fully aware of the reality of the situation, those caring for the child try to protect the child from a truth that they consider too difficult and painful to cope with by avoiding it in conversation, justifying it as the price to pay for an imaginary better future or, despite the obvious state of affairs, blatantly denying it.[20]

Such a widespread and destructive inability to communicate with children about death is due in great part to our received cultural visions of the good death: free from suffering, predicated on conscious, rational choice, and autonomous. This vision is the aim not only of advocates for euthanasia but also of palliative therapeutic models that emphasize acceptance. Focusing on conscious choice as the primary criterion for dying well has troubling implications for how we evaluate the death of children, whose capacity for autonomy is unclear.

How did we get here? I offer here a broad overview of the story. As I mentioned in the introduction, the context of death has changed substantially, most notably because of the rise of the medicalized death in the past century. Whereas care for the dying was once the role of the church and community, "medicine has become a social apparatus for the control of the dying."[21] Between 1945 and 1995, deaths occurring in Western European and North American hospitals rose from 40 percent to 90 percent.[22] This medicalized death not only changed the location of death from the home to the hospital, but brought to the scene its own interpretation of illness and death, namely the conviction that death is meaningless. As Jeffrey Bishop explains, "In viewing death exclusively as the destruction of meaning, medicine has aimed to do more than alleviate suffering: without realizing it, medicine hides death with technology and dissolves death in discourses."[23] This means that medicalized dying is characterized by the effort to avoid death—the "dying role" is replaced by the "sick role."[24]

Changes in the context of dying were accompanied by a change in attitude. Death became a depersonalized medical event, something that happens to a person, who is passive in the face of biological inevitability. This is in contrast to the perspective of the medieval *ars moriendi*, manuals that aimed to help the dying spiritually prepare for meeting God.[25] While the manuals supplicate against sudden death, what was once feared has now become the desired end: We pray that we may be lucky enough to die instantaneously, so the knowledge of our death does not come before death itself. We long for "a swift and sharp transition from vigorous existence to nonexistence."[26] Some scholars note that this cultural view of an ideal death is powerful enough that it has become the norm even among Christians. The dying process is no longer seen as "a stage of life that can both express and shape important personal commitments as well as strengthen key social and familial bonds."[27] Instead, it is widely accepted that there is no meaning to be found in the dying process.

But with a change of location and philosophy, medicalized death developed its own understanding of the good death. If first prize goes to the avoidance of death and dying entirely, the consolation prize is rational, conscious choice. Autonomy has come to dominate not only our medical system but also our moral imagination about death: "Conscious choice is the central aspect of being human for those of us living in the West, and it is the deciding feature of the good death."[28] It is worth noting that here meaning is found specifically in the act of conscious choice, not in death and dying themselves, which remain meaningless. Bishop finds this focus not only in advocacy for euthanasia, but also in therapeutic models that focus on acceptance. In the same way that medicine tries to fix the dying body, "medicine can attempt to "fix" the psychological wound, the sense of what is lost in death."[29] This fix, however, is stripped of substantive content: hope is no longer found in eternal life, or in God, but in the therapeutic process itself. In both models, what is on offer is control over the process of dying.

While practices *in situ* are more varied, this approach can be seen in pediatrics as well. Brian Carter's pediatric palliative care handbook places the role of helping children and family find meaning and purpose in dying in the hands of psychosocial team members—and that is all the entire book has to say on the subject.[30] Instead, it focuses on therapeutic models to help children and families *accept* the reality of death, for the implicit goal of these models is to move people from whatever emotions they are experiencing to acceptance. Most importantly for this chapter, what is central to the therapeutic model is the notion that acceptance must be freely chosen.

Our ideas of the good death are strongly related to how we approach the issue of suffering. At the beginning of *God, Medicine, and Suffering*, Stanley Hauerwas suggests that it is not suffering itself that makes us afraid, but rather the idea of pointless suffering. As Hauerwas notes, "Childhood suffering bothers us so deeply because we assume that children lack a life story which potentially gives their illness some meaning. In that respect I suspect we often fail to appreciate the richness of their young world as well as their toughness and resilience."[31] This is especially true when it comes to the death of children. As DeVries poignantly explains,

> We live by . . . the common assumption, or pretense, that human existence is "good" or "matters" or has "meaning," a glaze of charm or humor by which we conceal from one another and perhaps even ourselves the suspicion that it does not . . . Nowhere does this function more than in precisely such a slice of hell as a Children's Pavilion, where the basic truths would seem to mock any state of mind other than rage and despair.[32]

If death and the dying process are meaningless, then the suffering that is associated with them is also meaningless. Furthermore, in light of the emphasis on the conscious good death, suffering is reinterpreted: Meaning is not found in suffering, death and dying, but only in rational, conscious choice. What then is the good death? It is one that excludes children.

If we accept this conclusion, then the suffering at the end of a child's life becomes an impenetrable monolith we call "child suffering," a hopelessness to shield them from at all costs. This lack of meaning in dying and death makes the wholesale seeking after cure the only rational choice, because that gives a purpose to the suffering. The image of the child as a fighter, who does not give up to the very last breath, performs the same task. On the other hand, the exclusion of dying children out of concerns that they cannot understand, and that their suffering is meaningless, has a direct impact on the quality of end-of-life care offered to children. When we try to address the suffering of children with life-limiting illness, we are in a double bind: We waste too much breath lamenting the suffering of children and pay too little attention to their experiences of suffering, both physical and psycho-spiritual.

We have Freud and Piaget to thank for thinking that communicating about death and dying with young children is useless: "They asserted that young children know nothing about death and did not give it any thought."[33] The main reason for this belief was their overemphasis on the rational: They thought that concepts of death and resulting grief were only possible when one achieved a level of abstract reasoning. But children often communicate through stories, imagery, and play—they use media outside of formal reason. A toddler does not need to grasp the abstract concept of death in order to have ideas about it, or to grieve. Even preverbal infants are capable of feeling closeness and affection, and depend on it, in the midst of medical procedures and the dying process.[34]

Most initial studies looking at children's understanding of death were conducted among healthy children, who had little exposure to, or experience of, dying. More recent studies among dying children indicate that even very young children "know about their own death and can express this knowledge."[35] It is worth noting that we learned of children's ability to know about death when we took the time to actually talk to them, and to see value in imagination, stories, and play-acting as expressions of their knowledge. But despite the increasing number of studies demonstrating children's knowledge of their death and dying, it remains a common view that children, especially those under the age of ten, are unable to understand death and should be protected from any knowledge about it. This view excludes children from the conversation.

Thus, we have strikingly little information about the experience of death and dying among children, from infants to adolescents.[36] Of the studies that exist, most are retrospective and address only parents and health-care professionals, understandably excluding the dead child, but less defensibly excluding the insights of siblings and friends. But few (nonretrospective) studies even attempt to discuss with children their experiences, what causes them distress, how their symptoms are managed, or a variety of other factors that influence their dying. For example, in one study, the median age of the patients was 8.9, and some 20 percent of the children were still interactive and alert in the last day of life, not to mention the week leading up to the last day, which was also covered in the study, but the researchers did not talk to them.[37] Physical suffering is a key concern at end of life, but there is little data on the nature of this suffering, and therefore few resources to address it. Helping children die a good death "is complicated by a serious lack of data, as details of the last hours or weeks of a dying child's or adolescent's life are largely unknown."[38]

We know little, too, about what children think about prognostic openness—that is, communication that they will soon die. The 2021 article mentioned in the introduction, which found no change over time in the number of parents who communicated openly with their dying children, was based purely on retrospective data. There is thus a gap in knowledge. We know that many children are aware of their imminent death and attempt to communicate this. We know also that children often initiate conversations about death, and that many children find comfort in these conversations.[39]

Families and medical caregivers report that lack of communication around death increases distress for children who are dying, and it is correlated with long-term psychological morbidity in parents and siblings.[40] But we know almost nothing about how children themselves feel about open communication at the end of life, or about their own views of the distress caused by lack of communication, poor communication, or overcommunication. This is crucial information to learn, because the position in pediatric ethics at the end of life has been that open communication is not always best but should be decided on a case-by-case basis. This approach may indeed be correct, but we should certainly find out if it is effective from the perspective of the dying child, and not only their family.

The consequences of this lack of research are compounded by a small sample size. The decrease in child mortality, especially among the middle and upper classes, over the last century has allowed our culture to ignore the reality of child mortality and to pretend that it does not happen. Ulrika Kreicbergs argues that seriously ill children, their parents, and their medical team pay the price for the decrease in child mortality.[41] She singles out inadequate access to pediatric palliative care, as well as lack of data on how and where children die, and factors that affect whether they die a good death. The small sample size also means that much of what guides policy about dying children is adult-driven. For example, in a systematic review of research on where children want to die, Bluebond-Langner, et al. note that although many policy documents claim that children want to die at home, these assertions rely on adult-driven data.[42]

This inadequate research is also affected by the primacy of protection over participation in most approaches to children's rights and child research, and the mistaken idea that protection is possible without participation. This makes it very difficult to undertake research with dying children that does not have clear benefit, where benefit is defined primarily by a cure-seeking medical model. Although the UNCRC finally added participation rights of children in 1989, many research ethics guidelines on child research do not refer specifically to that document. Furthermore, most research ethics boards are guided by national policies that do not sufficiently differentiate issues specific to children. Perhaps most crucially, children are not consulted on these national policies and resulting research ethics guidelines.[43]

Sometimes these silences are understandable; children at end of life may be unable to communicate and some, as in the case of infants or children with developmental delay, are unable to answer questions. Children often die in pediatric intensive care units and, if there, are most likely to be ventilated and sedated.[44] There is also understandable concern about the vulnerability of children at the end of life, and the wish to protect them from further stress. But it clear that this lacuna in research on death and dying denies children a voice with respect to what they envision as the good death and hampers our ability to address the end-of-life concerns of those who are dying.

This lack of research can also obscure cultural factors that lead to different levels of care among children from different racial, economic, or geographical backgrounds.[45] Susan Derrington highlights the distressing finding in a major United States study that "Black children were about 20 percent less likely than white children to receive opioids and/or sedatives during their final days." She also reports that children who die in children's hospitals frequently receive better symptom management, especially pain management, at end of life. Cultural differences, which exist even among people who share the same religious beliefs or members of the same cultural background who belong to different religions, are also crucial to take into account in communications between health-care professionals and families. Most health-care professionals report feeling unprepared to deal with different cultural expressions, whether of grief, of physician-family relationships, or of decision-making, among other things.[46]

But there are other reasons not specific to medical treatment that make it difficult to attend to the voices of children at the end of life. Children are silenced by the denial of death and the common charade that we will all live forever.[47] The denial of the death of children is particularly potent, because childhood functions as a cultural image of future hope, to such an extent that childhood and death appear to be antitheses. The taboo of death in contemporary Western culture contributes to the geographic and social isolation of children, as they frequently die in hospital, often far away from their communities and separated from their friends and families.[48] It also contributes to the paucity of resources for guiding children and families at the end of life, and of cultural spaces where they are welcome. A colleague told me that what was hardest about the death of her child was the incredible silence she faced through the inability of those around her—friends, family, colleagues—to face this reality. Furthermore, many parents want to protect their healthy children from exposure to illness and death and are loath to let them visit a dying friend.[49]

There is a link, too, between the taboo of death and the unwillingness of parents to discuss death with dying children and adolescents. Children and adolescents are often excluded from visiting the sick and dying, and from the process of coming to terms with the death of a family member or of an acquaintance. We often keep children out of funerals and shield them from death, to the point that some churches have banned children from attending funerals.[50] This is especially problematic because talking about the death of a loved one is a key way parents and children are able to talk about the impending death of the child or young person.[51] In Verhey's words, "Where death is unmentionable, it is difficult to learn to die well."[52] The fact that we engage in this charade, with its expectation that grief and mourning be suppressed, denies children the opportunity to lament, rage, and express negative reactions to their illness and impending death.

Thus, children are frequently silenced by the inability of those around them to face death. This silence is often literal: Once their attempts to communicate knowledge about their death are rebuffed, children cease to bring it up. Dietrich Niethammer describes his experience with an adolescent patient who, after finding those around her were unwilling to address her death, stopped talking altogether in the last months of her life.[53] Referencing Bluebond-Langner's finding that parents spend less time with their children the closer they are to death, Hauerwas explains, "Our inability to be with our children in their deaths, an inability that results in our children dying alone, is but the result of our inability to deal with our own deaths."[54] Some parents even listed their child talking about dying as a symptom of most concern at end of life.[55] This avoidance of death strips both adults and children of their ability to explore their feelings: "As a result of the protectiveness [against death], our attitudes often deny us our humanness and strip us of our basic rights to discuss, explore, and share our feelings."[56] Furthermore, it can deny children the opportunity to talk about death, and to prepare for it, as well as blocking them from the opportunity to voice what is of concern to them, or to voice negative emotions and receive comfort.

Furthermore, access to palliative care, which not only helps families prepare for death but also has expertise in symptom control, often depends on the ability of parents to face death. Insufficient symptom management creates its own silences: Pain makes it hard to join in activities or to be with others; dyspnea steals breath needed to talk. "Referrals [to palliative care] typically are too few and late in the disease trajectory. Physicians tend to refer families to palliative care only if they think the family is willing or able to deal somewhat openly with their child's impending death."[57] The result is that these referrals usually come within the last day of a child's life. But the fact that physicians often only bring up palliative care if they perceive families to be sufficiently prepared is concerning, given that families have expressed the wish that their care team had discussed the option of including palliative care, especially for symptom management, with them sooner.[58]

The death of a child brings about the breakdown of relationships. Even before it arrives, the specter of death alienates us from ourselves, our normal lives, and our communities. This is intensified by the medicalization of dying, which "prematurely alienate[s] people from their own bodies, from their communities, and from God."[59] Serious illness and the dying process tear families apart, as they are overcome with anger, guilt, and an inability to communicate. Children are taken from their familiar surroundings—home, school, community life—and placed into an alien territory, the hospital. Parents, usually mothers, face an enormous series of pressures, exacerbated by the increased isolation from family and community support.[60] This is compounded when there are not outlets for parents and children to talk about what is going on in their lives, and by delayed involvement of palliative care, which can provide more support to address many of these issues.[61]

In the face of these breakdowns of relationship, it is easy to see how children are silenced. New environments are often overwhelming for healthy children, let alone a sick child. Children frequently feel responsibility for the disruption of family life as a result of their illness, and so feel significant pressure to be as perfect as possible in response, or to protect and comfort their parents. When children perceive that parents and health-care professionals are lying to them, they are less likely to open up and share what they are feeling. In short, all the normal support systems for a child have been disrupted.

This silencing also has an effect on those around the dying child. Over and over again, the literature shows that there is not just inadequate support for dying children, but for the siblings, families, and health-care professionals who care for them.[62] Siblings, who do not receive the focus that is on the child with life-limiting illness, are even more likely to be excluded from conversations about prognosis, and from meaningful participation in decision-making. Medical staff often feel inexperienced and unprepared for communicating about end-of-life care, or transition to palliative care. Health-care professionals too can have trouble accepting death, and this can affect use of adequate pain relief at the end of life. Other health-care professionals simply report being undertrained with respect to end-of-life care. Physicians and nurses also report the need to debrief and share stories around after the death of a patient, particularly in difficult cases.[63] Medical systems are also often ill-prepared for families from cultural backgrounds where decision-making is more spread out among a wide network of kin and community. To properly support those who face the suffering of children, to make meaning with them, to talk about death with them, requires large-scale support that is absent in our society.

Thus, it should be clear that I write none of this to blame parents, families, and health-care providers. The exact opposite, in fact! Those who surround dying children do so amid a culture that provides little space and support for them. My points are these: First, that we cannot expect children to die well, nor their loved ones to support them well, if we constantly pretend as a society that children do not die. Second, that there is no generic mono-lith that we can call "child suffering" that inevitably happens at the end of life. We have many concrete solutions to much of children's suffering. We can improve cultural spaces for families with sick children. We can seek to better train health-care professionals in conversations they feel unprepared for (pediatric hospitals already strive to do this and do a good job). We can reconsider our approach to research regarding dying children, and children in general. Once we stop avoiding child death, we can confront it. But to do so, we need to communicate with children, and together reject the idea that a good death is about control through rational autonomy. This is no easy task, and it does not remove the tragedy of child death. But as I will discuss in the next section, when we attend to children, we will find that they make meaning at the end of life.

✶✶✶

Children reveal that meaning can be made in the dying process, and that dependence and lack of control are not the destruction of our humanity we often think they are. In fact, children express their humanity beautifully without control. Confronting idealized adult-oriented conceptions of the good death and attending to children's ability to understand and confront death also help us to address the many sources of suffering at the end of a child's life. While it does not erase the tragedy and pain of child death, the knowledge that children can die well should help families and caregivers be able to face that death and make appropriate care decisions. When we communicate with children as they are dying, it is more likely that we can meet their needs. Most of all, by challenging conceptions of death and dying as meaningless, we can open ourselves to witnessing the meaning that children do make at the end of life.

In their insight into their experiences, in their creative ethical intentionality, and in meaning-making, children who are dying have much to teach us. Elisabeth Kübler-Ross, for one, was greatly influenced by children. In response to an interview question about what we need to face our fear of death, she states the need for a mature spiritual quadrant.[64] Although this may sound like the praise of adult rationality at first blush, what Kübler-Ross draws on, what MacDonald illustrates, and what I think is true of children, is that a mature spiritual quadrant does not necessarily rely on age and rationality, but on a multiplicity of meaning and on faith—something children often have in abundance. As Kübler-Ross writes,

> There are thousands of children who know death far beyond the knowledge adults have. Adults may listen to these children and shrug it off; they may think that children do not comprehend death; they may reject their ideas. But one day they may remember these teachings, even if it is only decades later when they face "the ultimate enemy" themselves. Then they will discover that those little children were the wisest of teachers, and they, the novice pupils.[65]

This point is not meant to instrumentalize the death of children, but rather to expand on what has been discussed already in this project: that our subjectivity is influenced by those around us, that children create meaning we do not expect, that they challenge us, teach us, and expand our sense of the world. This is no less true in their death.

Because we, children included, are relational and intersubjective beings, a good death is characterized by presence, by ongoing relationship with those whom we love. A good death is also characterized by silence, but a different kind than that discussed in the previous section. There is silence that annihilates—illness and suffering can take away our ability to speak, to know what to say, to receive comfort from words—but there is also good silence, a patient communication without words. One silence destroys meaning, the other allows for a plurality of meaning. Diamond becomes quieter after his first experience with the North Wind, a contemplative quiet that opens him to the needs of others. For many people, touch is a type of care and comfort that transcends words, and for some families, physical communication may be more appropriate than verbal communication.[66] This is most clearly illustrated by how we care for infants, for whom verbal explanations and reasons have little meaning, but who respond to a soothing touch.

Being present with those who are dying is about ongoing relationship, relationships which, because they are between people, are inherently meaningful. Children and adults exist in relationships as parents, aunts, uncles, sons, daughters, niblings, and more. In direct contrast to the obsession with autonomy in modern secular society, "participation in the family as an intimate association is one important way in which individuals find or construct meaning in their lives."[67] This cannot be a solo task, nor a task borne by parents alone. Instead, we should encourage the creation and maintenance of relational bonds within which the care of a child can be shared, by friends and family, by communities, and by health-care professionals. The relationship between children, their families, and health-care professionals is crucial to facilitating a good death for children and adolescents, and a trusting relationship between families and physicians provides the foundation for broaching difficult topics like prognosis and do not resuscitate orders in a way that families do not perceive as the care team giving up on their child. And sometimes adults must be willing to step out of the way and let children serve each other as comfort and support; other children can help children work through their grief in ways adults cannot.[68] The presence of other people is crucial for the dying process.

While the silence of presence is important, we must also be willing to listen to and speak honestly with children. Children, especially those with ongoing illness who are familiar with the hospital setting, are quite capable of grasping the fact that they are dying, even at a young age. This should come as no surprise; as I illustrated in the previous chapter, children come to know by experience, understanding, and reason, so it makes sense that children who have spent a long time being ill and dying know a lot about it. Even if their understanding of death is incomplete, we know that young children fear death, and toddlers are capable of grief at the death of someone they know, so they must grasp at least key elements of its meaning.[69] Children are often keen to share this knowledge, and frequently initiate communication about dying.[70] Many times, even young children understand that the only end to their suffering is the end of their life, and they are ready for it. Children also like to make plans for their death. Much like adults, children care that Christmas presents are purchased, and family gatherings planned. They may have visions about what they want their grave to look like, or to arrange who will care for their favorite possessions.[71]

Listening to children and being willing to discuss their experience is crucial to pain and symptom management, an essential practical element in the good death. On a practical level, this means conducting research on the symptoms that most distress children near the end of life, and it requires trusting children to be able to communicate their experiences. This trust is frequently lacking. Margaret Mohrmann tells the story of when, as a medical student, she was annoyed with a teenage patient named Milly who wheeled up and down the hallway complaining that her pain control was inadequate, despite the fact that her dosing and schedule was exactly what was recommended. After a few weeks of this, and after some prompting from her supervisor, Mohrmann "saw, with great clarity, that [she] could talk to Milly about her pain and its control," leading to the creation of a pain management dosage and schedule that actually relieved Milly's symptoms.[72] Not only was Milly more comfortable, but she was able to spend time with other children and socialize with the nurses, something she was previously unable to do. Listening to children means attending to the ways they communicate, like play-acting and other creative means or, as in the case of Milly, in manners downright annoying to adults. Being open to all these methods of communication allows us to properly attend to the issues that particularly concern children.

Stories and fantasy are an especially potent way for children and adults to communicate together about death. Through nonsense (in the face of the mystery and unintelligibility of death), storytelling, presence, relationship, and dependence, children model the good death. Through these ways we can speak honestly with children about their pain, loneliness, and sorrow, allow them to freely express their suffering, and offer them comfort. We receive and create these stories about the meaning of life, of childhood, and of death *together* and through the witness of children, who have much to teach us about confronting and overcoming the sources of suffering at the end of life. In so many creative ways, children make meaning in the dying process.

Stories give us words where there are no words. They depict endless possibilities of encounter and response. Through story, we can put on, as it were, the character of another. Through talking about storylines or about challenges a character faces, children can indicate their own fears and hopes. If Hauerwas is right that one of the reasons we find the death of children so tragic is that we worry they do not have the capacity to create a narrative that gives meaning to their lives,[73] then it is my position that this concern not only overlooks the incredible capacities for creating narratives, real and fantastical, that children do have, but also ignores the role of *shared* stories, of telling stories to children, and of encouraging them to tell stories. Children are able to learn and explore who they are through story. This bears out in research among dying children and their families, where fairy tales and fantasy stories are one of the main vehicles for discussing death.[74]

One example is the popularity of the children's book *Charlotte's Web* among dying children. Ladd and Kopelman suggest a number of reasons for this: The dying character is central to the plot, the main character is a runt saved from being culled, and Charlotte listens to Wilbur's fears about death and comforts him. Further, children may recognize their own experiences in the symptoms expressed by the failing Charlotte.[75] But the power of stories goes far beyond one book. A 2015 study found that fairy tales were the most common vehicle for discussion about death between parents and dying children, regardless of age.[76] The authors note that fairy tales allowed parents and children to enter into a discussion about death without specifically addressing death, and so provided a way into a conversation that might otherwise have been too difficult.[77] Children are able to find meaning in these narratives, seeing a correspondence between these stories and their own experience. Similarly, stories often tell the truth otherwise denied to children; to arrive at the back of the North Wind, Diamond must pass through her, something she tells him honestly will hurt him.[78]

However, I believe that stories, and especially fairy tales, do more than simply facilitate discussions about death. Fairy tales allow for and encourage a multiplicity of meaning, a slippage between the imminent and transcendent. They are liminal stories, caught between the real world we experience and are familiar with, and a magical realm, often outside of time and the rules of physics. These stories tie together death and meaning in a way our culture does not understand: In the nonsense poetry Diamond creates after his first experience at the back of the North Wind, he plays with multiple meanings of a word, creates relationships between things that do not naturally connect, exaggerates ideas or events to an extreme, and takes figurative language as literal, all of which help his readers to think about death differently than predominant cultural attitudes.[79]

Diamond's lighthearted take on death, while it doesn't destroy meaning, relieves some of the fear associated with it, though without making false promises, like the absence of pain. This play with multiplicity can show us that there is plenty of meaning to be found in death and dying. Society's good death demands control and a rational explanation that will satisfy. But this does not exist. Children see more clearly than adults that death is a mystery, but this does not mean meaning is absent. Fairy tales also express faith in the existence of this other realm—a faith adults often find much harder to hold on to. For MacDonald, "because death has been defeated, because it teaches one to enjoy life, it is something that can finally be accepted."[80] Stories help adults cope with death, too.[81] Fairy tales transcend age categories, and are embodiments of hope.

If it is fairy tales and nonsense poetry that allow us to take death lightly and to play with a multiplicity of meaning, it is lament that allows us to take it seriously, to name that which destroys and to grieve its effects. We must be ready to hear children's anger, the sense of injustice, sorrow, and pain: This is both theologically and clinically appropriate. We know from clinical experience that "the terminally ill child is reported to grieve loss of function and future and to worry about being forgotten, experiencing pain, and leaving family members behind in sorrow."[82] We know too, as Verhey writes, that "we may . . . learn from Christ in Gethsemane that, in the face of death, it is fitting to lament, to cry out to God, to ask that we be spared from death."[83] A counterpart to MacDonald's approach to death in *At the Back of the North Wind* is found in his *Diary of an Old Soul*, where he, with great difficulty and grief, "attempts to reimagine death, acknowledging its hideousness and horror whilst trying to understand it as a spiritual rebirth."[84] Lament tells the story of pain and suffering in the context of relationship with God and with others.

Failure to acknowledge this suffering of children, and the hideousness and horror that can and often does accompany their death, will lead to less humane treatment for them. Addressing suffering means being willing to listen to children, to comfort them, and to give them hope. It may also require us to sacrifice our own notions about protecting our children from the realities of the world, and instead allow them to participate in their own care. Addressing suffering and hearing lament also enables the creation of meaning in the dying process, as children and their families reflect on what they mean to each other, on what they value, and on the ever-variegated experiences of love. Many of MacDonald's fairy tales illustrate the ways in which joy is impossible without sorrow. To learn about sorrow in all its forms is then to learn, to prepare the ground for, hitherto unknown joy.

This childlike witness to the intergenerational connection and meaning-making that can occur through story reveals something about our shared humanity. Stories allow us to hold together disparate and contradictory ideas, the tragic and the beautiful together. Stories that hold together multiple meanings and paths can also help to overcome the dichotomy between "fighting the disease" and "giving up on the child." This, then, may help families integrate palliative care earlier, even as they hope that the disease prognosis will change.[85] Stories also allow flexibility that reasoning and guidelines do not. Stories make space for the many varying and sometimes contradictory meanings of death and dying. Characters can embody multiple characters and roles. Stories open up the possibility that there are multiple paths to take to the same place. When we attend to children, we can note trends and commonalities. But children's response to death and dying in individual circumstances transcend statistics. Nor does a child have to die in an idealized manner to make meaning, to be loved, and to be in relationship with God and those around them. There is space at the deathbed for lament, anger, and confusion, as much as there is for hope and love.

Once we accept this multiplicity of meanings, we can confront the cultural view that death and dying are meaningless, and any hope for a good death comes from the ability to make conscious choices around death, both in treatment options and in our control of our own narrative. Many who study child death demonstrate that children are often better than adults at facing and accepting death. Research among children at the end of life shows that children are much less likely to ask questions about the meaning of suffering, or to ask questions of "why me?" That is, children are less likely to focus on the existential questions of suffering, but focus on the concrete realities of their situation.[86] Most models of acceptance exclude children based on a narrow account of reason, but younger children, who are used to not being in control of their lives, may find acceptance easy because they are not holding on to control, and because they do not fully grasp the permanence of death. We should not discount their acceptance but seek to learn from it.

Stories also allow for a creative reevaluating of societal roles. In the phenomenon of mutual pretense described by Bluebond-Langner, one of the key contributing factors was that, in the face of death, the roles of parents and child were no longer valid.[87] She attributes this to the adult-oriented goals of childhood. Children are selected and groomed to be successful adults; there is in North American culture a clear desire for "perfect" children who will grow to fulfill the demands of a market economy.[88] Because there was no meaning of this kind in the lives of children who were not going to grow up, both parents and children simply pretended that the children were not dying; this pretense allowed both children and parents to fulfill their societal roles, although they were no longer valid. Aware that they were dying, some children "felt they could not speak freely, even with people they trusted, about their awareness of the prognosis."[89] Cultural ideals about children and the dominance of adult-oriented goals obscure opportunities for meaning-making in the dying process.

Of course, there is nothing inherently wrong with continuing many aspects of life for children with life-limiting illnesses; continued opportunities to go to school, learn instruments, and participate in other pursuits often help children to maintain a sense of purpose and self-confidence. It is not wrong, certainly, that when children are dying, we are overcome with pain not only at the loss of their presence now but the loss of what they could become: seeing them age, become our friends, find careers they are passionate about, fall in love, have children of their own, and so on. These hopes and dreams for the future are not wrong and are deeply part of who we are as people. The danger occurs when we solely fixate on these future visions. Seeing children as a practice ground for a real humanity found in the future devalues children's current experiences and robs them of the ability to make meaning out of their present life. There is a difference between mourning a lost future and despairing over a present rendered "meaningless" because it has no future. Furthermore, believing that children have nothing to offer in the present is a self-fulfilling prophecy: We then fail to see or hear the richness of the experiences of children and young people.

In opposition to adult-oriented criteria of value, Mercer argues that children are divine gifts that we steward, not own; we do not choose who is given to us, and we do not control the length of time for which they are given. As Mercer explains, we must understand that children are divine gifts even when they do not *look* like gifts—even when they are messy, dirty, demanding, difficult, and, I would add, dying.[90] Children are gifts as children, not as potential adults, not as the hope for our future. A Christian understanding of children and their dying cannot start with the goal of "growing up." If growing up is the goal, then children are nothing more than a means to the desired end: at best, a person capable of self-determination; at worst, an opportunity for parents to fulfill their own dreams. Instead, we must recognize that children are intersubjective and relational beings who impact our lives from the moment of their conception and whose value is that they exist in relationship to others and to God. Those who die as children are not failures, but rather "childhood [is located] within God's eternity—not as a phase to be outgrown and left behind, but also as an eternal feature of humanity."[91] There is a difference between acknowledging the ideal, or even normal, continuum of a child's life, and ascribing inherent value to that ideal only.

The appropriateness of reevaluating these societal roles is not simply a nice idea, but emerges from observing the behavior of children with life-limiting illness. Children step into roles as teachers and caregivers, forming moral approaches to the pain and suffering of their parents and siblings. Margaret Mohrmann tells the story of Luke, a young boy of five who was ready for death, knowing that it was the only end to his suffering. But Luke's mother was not ready. Knowing this, and not wanting to disturb his mother who was sleeping peacefully beside his bed, he crept off to the bathroom and died there so that he would not disturb her.[92] Similarly, after his first experience at the back of the North Wind, Diamond gains a new ability to recognize when others are miserable, knows how to alleviate their misery, and protects the innocent.[93] Children at the end of life want to care for their families, and even use their final weeks and months to care for the needs and wishes of others.

It means that all of us who are responsible for raising and nurturing children—meaning parents and grandparents, but also extended families, churches, municipalities, and all those who share in the cultural and moral environment of a child—have a role to play in creating and sharing our own stories around death. It is worth repeating Hugh Brody's words from the introduction to this book: "The human mind depends on speaking and listening, hearing and telling stories. If there is silence, then there is much about who we are that we cannot know. Silence in the home can leave a void in a child."[94] Silence at the deathbed can do the same. It can leave a void in the child who is dying, but also in their siblings and friends, families, and caregivers. While children often communicate knowledge about their death and make meaning through stories, it is equally true that children often rely heavily on parents, caregivers, and loved ones to communicate prognoses and for strength and support to cope.[95]

In the fostering of relationships, in the creation of new stories, and in providing cultural space for those who are dying, grieving, and bereaved, the church has an important role to play. It needs to be a place that receives the parents of dying children and provides them with a place to find both comfort and honesty. In welcoming those who care for dying children, we must be willing to take on some of their burden. Instead of being people who "conspire to hide our deaths from ourselves and from one another, calling our conspiracy 'respect for the individual,'"[96] as a church we should acknowledge that we are all created with limitations—from dust to dust—and that our completeness is found in God. The church should refuse the cultural taboo of death: "There can be no way to remove the loneliness of death of . . . children unless they see witnessed in the lives of those who care for them a confidence rooted in friendship with God and with one another."[97] The church also provides tools for the reparation of relationships. Children often understand their illness as a form of punishment; similarly, siblings may worry that something they did to a sibling caused the illness. Here, the sacrament of confession and absolution provides an opening to confront these concerns. This approach to death is something that should be enacted for everyone, not just for the dying. It is equally important to talk to children about death when they (and those they know) are *not* dying. That is, we should prepare children to welcome the dying and walk alongside them. And when they do, we should be prepared to learn from their example.

This chapter is not intended to be prescriptive about the right set of actions to take at the end of life, nor too directive about how communication at the end of life should be undertaken. As I said earlier, this chapter is not a clinical manual for health-care professionals. Nor is it a pastoral manual. Instead, it is an invitation to confront the cultural forces that prevent us from reimagining a child's deathbed. But no matter what concrete actions we take, we should be open and responsive to children's communication, and provide them with the resources to confront what they are going through, remembering that they are moral subjects and agents who are in relation with those around them, and extremely attentive to spoken and unspoken dynamics, to taboo topics and discomfort, and to silence. We must keep in mind that it has been repeatedly shown that children who are made aware of their diagnosis and prognosis do better.

I am, then, not recommending that every single family be forced into a standard model of open communication. What I am arguing for is responsiveness to children's own communication. Beyond that, I am advocating for a particular view of children as moral subjects and agents that implies certain things for adult communication with children. It is also an opportunity to talk with families who are reluctant to communicate with their children about their *reasons* for this reluctance. To gently point out that their child is communicating knowledge of the inevitable. To make space for children to exercise their moral subjectivity and agency. To invite others to consider why they are making their decisions, to invite them to ask their child if they want to be informed, and to lay out their vision of a child as moral subject/agent. They may simply never have thought about it. That is, in a pluralistic setting, we can still lay out our own vision and give others the opportunity to respond. We should study the culturally specific elements of children's ethical intentionality, so as to better meet them as moral subjects and agents in their own contexts.

But more than that, there is overwhelming evidence that children are both eager and able to discuss their knowledge of their own dying, both in direct ways and in indirect ways, such as expressing treatment preferences, planning their funerals, and disposing of their possessions. Some are not eager to discuss it—that is also fine, and certainly does not mean they cannot die well. Some children are, by culture and personality, indirect communicators. But because of children's ethical intentionality, in response to their desires to be included, and in response to their incredible capacity to make meaning, we should prioritize their participation over their protection, though this participation should be done appropriately for their preferences and stage of comprehension. We should speak openly with children for the same reasons we speak openly with adults: because they are moral subjects and agents who should be respected in their views. Child death is, in part, tragic not because we have failed some ideal of protected childhood, but because children are already competent and contributing members of society, even if we don't see it.

In all of these ways, there are many opportunities for meaningful encounter in the dying process. But to say that a child can die a good death is not to say that dying is peaceful, pain-free, or to be romanticized in any way. A good death is still a tragedy. Children, their families, and their care providers face innumerable griefs and challenges. A good death does not mean that they must bottle up their emotions and pretend that things are all right. And yet, even in that deep sorrow, there are opportunities for connection, comfort, even joy. But dying well is not easy, any more than it is easy for a child to live a good life among the many griefs and challenges of the world.

The reality is that attending to dying children is a mutual encounter. We need to attend to children to know how to best meet their needs, and they can teach us about the meaning they find in their own dying. But they rely significantly on those around them to support them. "Openness, respect, and truthfulness . . . between parents and their children . . . can contribute to deepening the experience, closeness, understanding of life, and confirmation of mutual affection."[98] So, then, hope that children will die a good death is found in who they are as human beings, in their relationships, in honest speech with them, in the endless possibilities for meaning-making present in our lives and deaths, in lament, and in mitigating the sources of suffering at the end of life. We need to stop avoiding and hiding child death, instead making space for it in human life. Only then will we be able to learn from children, and only then will we be able to help them to die well.

⁎

For Christians, the overarching story of eschatological hope brings meaning to death and dying. Eschatology has been a sore subject in a lot of child theology because of its adult-oriented nature, as I discussed in the first chapter. Eschatology has also sometimes enabled escapism from death; in certain eschatological views, death is eclipsed by the reality of the resurrection. But a properly childist eschatology is not one of escape from death, but one in which children are the goal of the Christian life.

As Christians, our hope for overcoming suffering and death is not that it is "natural" or that "we can learn from it." Addressing the suffering of children means seeing that suffering in the larger context of the gospel story: in Jesus's welcoming of children, in the suffering of Christ on the cross, and in the hope of the resurrection. In the end, our hope is not found even in each other, except for in the ways in which all human meaning, relationships, and love find their wholeness in God. We are intersubjective beings, we share meaning-making, and we continue to share in that even after we die.[99] But, at the same time, we should not make the mistake of focusing on the deathbed to the exclusion of all else. Like MacDonald, we must stretch out our hands in childlike trust, "beyond death into the presence of God."[100]

This is the context in which death can be both lamented and accepted. Verhey argues against a commendation of death, saying that death is never a liberation, never a friend to be welcomed, but "is a tyrant to be defeated."[101] But why can it not be both? Did Jesus not transform death into a pathway to life? Thus it is both to be feared and welcomed, lamented and celebrated; in his *Diary*, MacDonald understood death both in physical terms with all its horror and grief, and "as a spiritual awakening, a final ordeal before the soul's reunion with the divine."[102] Death for MacDonald was the great equalizer, not, like in the poems of *Death and the Lady*, by lowering those of high standard, but by raising all people to brotherhood and sisterhood in Christ. If our hope lies in the resurrection and life in the Spirit, then death is the only way to resurrection; the only way to the back of the North Wind is through it.

Our selves and our relationships find wholeness in God, the very same God who raised Jesus from the dead and promised that he is but the first fruits of the resurrection.

> That hope, Jesus's hope, the hope we share by the gift of the Spirit, was cosmic in its scope. . . . [But not] less personal by being cosmic. Each Christian hopes for the good future of God—and to share in it. We may hope to participate in the resurrection of Christ. We may hope for "the redemption of our bodies" (Rom 8:23) along with the renewal of the whole creation, in solidarity with both Christ and any who weep because the future is not yet.[103]

We should hope for a good death and do what we can to bring it about; we should work hard to reduce the pain and distress of dying children and their families. But it is not the locus of our hope.

Rather, at all stages, the locus of our hope is that we remain children of God, loved by God, in whom our completeness is found. "The fullness of childhood consists in being children of God."[104] To die is to enter into eschatological childhood, as Rahner puts it. Ultimately, Christians find their hope in the resurrection. This resurrection is not the erasure of our lives on earth, nor some hope for an adult-oriented future, but rather the fulfillment of who we are: children of God. In this way, rather than providing us with a way to escape the present, eschatological hope promises us that all our present actions find meaning in God's future. Our completeness must always and can only be found in God, and in understanding this, death can be befriended. In understanding this, we can testify that children can die a good death.

NOTES

1 Manuel Jacinto Sarmento, Rita de Cássia Marchi, and Gabriela de Pina Trevisan, "Beyond the Modern 'Norm' of Childhood: Children at the Margins as a Challenge for the Sociology of Childhood" in *Theorising Childhood: Citizenship, Rights and Participation*, eds. Claudio Baraldi and Tom Cockburn (London: Palgrave MacMillan, 2018), 135–158. Some scholars refer to what I am calling "Western culture" as the Global North.

2 United Nations General Assembly, *Convention on the Rights of the Child*, November 20, 1989, United Nations, Treaty Series, vol. 1577.

3 Claudio Baraldi and Tom Cockburn, "Introduction: Lived Citizenship, Rights and Participation in Contemporary Europe" in *Theorising Childhood: Citizenship, Rights and Participation*, eds. Claudio Baraldi and Tom Cockburn (London: Palgrave MacMillan, 2018), 1–28.

4 George MacDonald, *George MacDonald and His Wife*, ed. Greville MacDonald (London: Johannesen Publishing, 1998), 524.

5 J. Patrick Pazdziora, "'The Path of Pain' George MacDonald's Portrayal of Death in The Diary of an Old Soul," *North Wind* 36 (2017): 97.

6 Charles Taylor, *Sources of the Self: The Making of the Modern Identity* (Cambridge: Harvard University Press, 1989), 13.

7 See, among others, Franca Benini, Roberta Vecchi, and Marcello Orzalesi, "A Charter for the Rights of the Dying Child," Correspondence, *The Lancet* 383 (2014): 1547–1548, Pamela S. Hinds, et al., "Key Factors Affecting Dying Children and Their Families," *Journal of Palliative Medicine* 8 (2005): 70–78; Li Jalmsell, et al., "On the Child's Own Initiative: Parents Communicate with Their Dying Child about Death," *Death Studies* 39 (2015): 111–117; Dietrich Niethammer, *Speaking Honestly with Sick and Dying Children & Adolescents: Unlocking the Silence*, trans. Victoria W. Hill (Baltimore: Johns Hopkins University Press, 2012).

8 Teens report losing friends because of their illness. M. Slaninka, P. Krajmer, A. Kolenova, "Main Topics Related to the Disease, Death, and Dying in Communication between Parents and Their Adolescent Children with Incurable Cancer," *Bratislava Medical Journal* 122 (2021): 572–576.

9 Jason Tans, "Playing for Time," *Wired* January 2016. https://www.wired.com/2016/01/that-dragon-cancer/

10 See summary in Nancy A. Contro, et al., "Hospital Staff and Family Perspectives Regarding Quality of Pediatric Palliative Care," *Pediatrics* 114 (2004): 1251.

11 Joyce Ann Mercer, *Welcoming Children: A Practical Theology of Childhood* (St. Louis: Chalice Press, 2005), 111.

12 "Top 10 Children's Books About Death and Dying," *Storyberries* 2013. https://tinyurl.com/nhd5822d.

13 Jen Baker, "Traditions and Anxieties of (Un)Timely Child Death in *Jude the Obscure*," *The Thomas Hardy Journal* 33 (2017): 61–84: Thomas W. Laqueur, *The Work of the Dead: A Cultural History of Mortal Remains* (Princeton: Princeton University Press, 2015).

14 See Slaninka, et al, "Main Topics"; Myra Bluebond-Langner, *The Private Worlds of Dying Children* (Princeton: Princeton University Press, 1980); Jalmsell, et al., "On the Child's Own Initiative."

15 Bluebond-Langner, *Private Worlds*, 223–225.

16 Slaninka, et al., "Main Topics," 574.

17 Jalmsell, et al., "On the Child's Own Initiative," 111.

18 Slaninka, et al., "Main Topics," 573.

19 Benini, et al., "A Charter for the Rights of the Dying Child"; Contro, et al., "Hospital Staff and Family Perspectives," 1248–1252; Hinds, et al., "Key Factors," 70–78; Ulrika Kreicbergs, "Why and Where Do Children Die," *Acta Pædiatrica* 107 (2018): 1671–1672; Niethammer, *Speaking Honestly with Sick and Dying Children & Adolescents.*

20 Franca Benini, et al., "A Charter," 1547–1548.

21 Jeffrey P. Bishop, *The Anticipatory Corpse: Medicine, Power, and the Care of the Dying* (Notre Dame: University of Notre Dame Press, 2011), 23.

22 Allen Verhey, *The Christian Art of Dying: Learning from Jesus* (Grand Rapids: Eerdmans, 2011); and Bishop, *The Anticipatory Corpse,* 13–14.

23 Bishop, *The Anticipatory Corpse,* 17.

24 Verhey, *Christian Art of Dying,* 14.

25 Verhey, *Christian Art of Dying,* 79–88. Cathleen Kaveny, *Law's Virtues: Fostering Autonomy and Solidarity in American Society* (Washington, DC: Georgetown University Press, 2012), 141–144.

26 Kaveny, *Law's Virtues,* 142.

27 Kaveny, 142; Stanley Hauerwas, *God, Medicine, and Suffering,* (Grand Rapids, MI: Eerdmans, 1990), 98.

28 Bishop, *Anticipatory Corpse,* 19.

29 Bishop, *Anticipatory Corpse,* 3.

30 Brian S. Carter, Marcia Levetown, and Sarah E. Friebert, eds., *Palliative Care for Infants, Children, and Adolescents: A Practical Handbook,* 2nd ed. (Baltimore: Johns Hopkins University Press, 2011), 206.

31 Hauerwas, *God, Medicine, and Suffering,* 67.

32 Peter DeVries, *The Blood of the Lamb,* quoted in Hauerwas, *God, Medicine, and Suffering,* 23.

33 Niethammer, *Speaking Honestly,* 101. For a prolonged discussion of Freud and Piaget's views, as well as their legacy, see chapter 8.

34 Myra Bluebond-Langner, et al., "Preferred Place of Death for Children and Young People with Life-Limiting and Life-Threatening Conditions: A Systematic Review of the Literature and Recommendations for Future Inquiry and Policy," *Palliative Medicine* 27 (2013): 711; Jalmsell, et al., "On the Child's Own Initiative," 114; Niethammer, *Speaking Honestly,* 12, 114.

35 Niethammer, 114.

36 Ulrika Kriecberg, "Why and Where do Children Die," *Acta Pædiatrica* 107 (2018): 1671; Bluebond-Langner et al., "Preferred Place of Death," 706; Hinds et al., "Key Factors," 71.

37 Ross Drake, Judy Frost, and John J. Collins, "The Symptoms of Dying Children" *Journal of Pain and Symptom Management* 26 (2003): 594–603.

38 Hinds et al., "Key Factors," 71.

39 Jalmsell et al., "On the Child's Own Initiative," 110–112. Niethammer, *Speaking Honestly*, Chapter 10.

40 Contro, et al., "Hospital Staff and Family Perspectives," 1248–1252; Jalmsell, "On the Child's Own Initiative," 112.

41 Ulrika Kreicbergs, "Why and Where Do Children Die," 1671.

42 Bluebond-Langner, et al., "Preferred Place of Death," 706.

43 Nancy Bell, "Ethics in Child Research: Rights, Reason and Responsibilities," *Children's Geographies* 6:1 (2008), 7–20.

44 Drake, et al., "Symptoms of Dying Children," 599.

45 Susan Derrington, "Are We Doing Right by Dying Children?" *The Journal of Paediatrics* 166 (2015): 525.

46 Contro, et al., "Hospital Staff and Family Perspectives," 1250.

47 Niethammer, *Speaking Honestly*, 36; Verhey, *Christian Art of Dying*, 11–16; see also Geoffrey Gorer's 1965 essay "The Pornography of Death."

48 Niethammer, *Speaking Honestly*, 37, 18.

49 Niethammer, *Speaking Honestly*, 40.

50 "Three articles mention cultural factors. Montel et al. state that 'In France, as in most Western countries, death is a subject of taboo' (32, 35). Nineteen of the 21 families in the study did not discuss impending death with the [children and young people]." Bluebond-Langner, et al., "Preferred place of death," 711; see also Niethammer, *Speaking Honestly*, 39. The banning of children from funerals was reported to me by a student who was also a minister in the Church of Scotland.

51 Jalmsell, et al., "On the Child's Own Initiative," 116; Niethammer, *Speaking Honestly*, 38.

52 Verhey, *Christian Art of Dying*, 16.

53 Bluebond-Langner, *Private Worlds*, 189; Niethammer, *Speaking Honestly*, xiii.

54 Hauerwas, *God, Medicine, and Suffering*, 146.

55 Michele Pritchard, et al., "Factors That Distinguish Symptoms of Most Concern to Parents from Other Symptoms of Dying Children," *Journal of Pain and Symptom Management* 39 (2010): 631.

56 Jo-Eileen Guylay, *The Dying Child* (Toronto: McGraw-Hill, 1978), ix.

57 Bluebond-Langner, et al., "Preferred Place of Death," 710.

58 Contro, et al., "Hospital Staff and Family Perspectives," 1249–1250.

59 Verhey, *Christian Art of Dying*, 173.

60 Guylay, *Dying Child*, 17, 35; Hinds, et al., "Key Factors," 70.

61 Drake, et al., "Symptoms of Dying Children," 595.

62 See, among others, Hinds, et al., "Key Factors," 70–78; Drake, et al., "Symptoms of Dying Children"; Contro, et al., "Hospital Staff and Family Perspectives," 1248–1252; Contro, et al., "Family Perspectives on the Quality of Pediatric Palliative Care," in *Arch Pediatr Asolesc Med* (2002): 14–19.

63 Lovisa Furingsten, Reet Sjögren, and Maria Forsner, "Ethical Challenges When Caring for Dying Children." *Nursing Ethics* 22 (2015): 184.

64 Elisabeth Kübler-Ross, interview with K. Kramer. Kenneth Kramer, "You Cannot Die Alone: Dr. Elisabeth Kübler-Ross (July 8, 1926–August 24, 2004)," *OMEGA - Journal of Death and Dying* 50 (2005): 83.

65 Elisabeth Kübler-Ross, *On Children and Death: How Children and Their Parents Can and Do Cope with Death* (New York: Touchstone Books, 1997), xii.

66 Jalmsell, et al., "On the Child's Own Initiative," 117.

67 Dan W. Brock and Allen E. Buchanan, *Deciding for Others: The Ethics of Surrogate Decision Making* (New York: Cambridge University Press, 1989), 136.

68 Guylay, *Dying Child*, 51.

69 Niethammer, *Speaking Honestly*, 108.

70 Jalmsell, et al., "On the Child's Own Initiative," 114. This study included children diagnosed between the ages of 0–17 (and who died under the age of 25) and found surprising correspondence in the ways children talked about death, especially the use of fairy tales, across all age groups.

71 Jalmsell, et al., "On the Child's Own Initiative," 115.

72 Margaret Mohrmann, *Attending Children: A Doctor's Education* (Washington, DC: Georgetown University Press, 2006), 26.

73 Hauerwas, *God, Medicine, and Suffering*, 146.

74 Jalmsell, et al., "On the Child's Own Initiative," 115.

75 Kopelman, "Charlotte the Spider," 123–126; Rosalind Ekman Ladd, "Death and Children's Literature: *Charlotte's Webb* and the Dying Child," in *Children and Health Care: Moral and Social Issues*, eds. Loretta M. Kopelman and John C. Moskop (Boston: Kluwer Academic Publishers, 1989), 108–113.

76 Jalmsell, et al., "On the Child's Own Initiative," 113.

77 Parents often expressed thankfulness for narratives "that made it easier to talk about death with their child." Jalmsell, et al., 115.

78 MacDonald, *At the Back*, 107.

79 Melody Green, "Death and Nonsense in the Poetry of George MacDonald's *At the Back of the North Wind* and Lewis Carroll's *Alice Books*." *North Wind* 30 (2011): 38.

80 Green, 47.

81 Furingsten, et al., "Ethical Challenges," 184.

82 Hinds, et al., "Key Factors," 71–72.

83 Verhey, *Christian Art of Dying*, 222.

84 Pazdziora, "The Path of Pain," 97.

85 Slaninka, et al., "Main Topics," 573.

86 Chris Feudtner, Jeff Haney, and Martha A. Dimmers, "Spiritual Care Needs of Hospitalized Children and Their Families: A National Survey of Pastoral Care Providers' Perceptions," *Pediatrics* 111 (2003): 69–70.

87 Bluebond-Langner, *Private Worlds*, 198–209.

88 Joyce Ann Mercer, *Welcoming Children: A Practical Theology of Childhood* (St. Louis: Chalice Press, 2005), 92–94. This utilitarian bend affects not only the consumer items we purchase, but also our medical decisions.

89 Bluebond-Langner, *Private Worlds*, 189.

90 Mercer, *Welcoming Children*, 245. See also Joel James Shuman and Brian Volck, "What are Children For?" in *On Moral Medicine: Theological Perspectives in Medical Ethics*, eds. Theresa M. Lysaught, Joseph Kotva, Stephen E. Lammers, and Allen Verhey (Grand Rapids: Eerdmans, 1998), 763.

91 Mercer, *Welcoming Children*, 252.

92 Mohrmann, *Attending Children*, 79–80.

93 Green, "Death and Nonsense," 41–42.

94 Hugh Brody, "'The Deepest Silences': What Lies behind the Arctic's Indigenous Suicide Crisis," *The Guardian*. July 21, 2022. https://tinyurl.com/2dk92rvn.

95 Slaninka, et al., "Main Topics," 573.

96 Hauerwas, *God, Medicine, and Suffering*, 101.

97 Hauerwas, *God, Medicine, and Suffering*, 148.

98 Slaninka, et al., "Main Topics," 573.

99 For a remarkable study on the ways in which the dead continue to influence the lives of the living in constructing cultural meaning, see Thomas Laqueur, *The Work of the Dead: A Cultural History of Mortal Remains* (Princeton: Princeton University Press, 2015).

100 Pazdziora, "The Path of Pain," 105.

101 Verhey, *The Christian Art of Dying*, 183.

102 Pazdziora, "The Path of Pain," 97.

103 Verhey, *The Christian Art of Dying*, 200.

104 Karl Rahner, "Ideas for a Theology of Childhood," in *Theological Investigations*, vol. 8, *Further Theology of the Spiritual Life 2*, trans. David Bourke (New York: Herder & Herder, 1971), 43.

CHAPTER 4

Does a Child Mean What She Says?

In the second chapter of this book, I argued that children are genuine moral agents who engage in the same moral world as adults, inherit moral language, imitate moral conduct, and play creatively with their moral environment. In the third chapter, I argued that children can and do make meaning in death, and that we ought to engage with children through open communication. And in both cases, I argued that children have something to teach us about the moral life in general, and about death and dying in particular. They open up horizons of human meaning and reveal aspects of our humanity that we have forgotten, ignored, or have yet to experience.

But to communicate openly with children, teach children moral reasoning, and especially to *listen* to children, we must assess whether children can meaningfully and truthfully express their experience. This chapter thus asks the question: *Does a child mean what she says?* That is, *Can we trust that what a child says is true to what she feels? Do children have sufficient rational capacity to meaningfully contribute to conversations? How do we make sense of children's penchant to mix fact and fantasy in their communication?* In this chapter, I will be talking about a child's ability to communicate both *meaningfully* and *accurately*, where the relationship between these two concepts depends on one's approach to language.

The belief that children are incapable of meaningfully and reliably communicating their experiences manifests itself in our culture in many ways. For example, scholars believe that a major reason why child sex abuse by authority figures often goes unexamined is the general assumption that children's expressions of their experiences are inherently unreliable. That is, there is a link between disbelief of child witnesses, and cultural views about children's grasp of concepts like sex, sexuality, and sexual abuse—a link that explains in part our failure to protect children. The assumption that children do not know what sex is contributes to disbelief when they describe abusive sexual experiences. This reaction is compounded by the belief that children lie more frequently and easily than adults, thus rendering their testimony less trustworthy.[1]

The adult tendency to dismiss children's utterances as unreliable or irrelevant on account of their immaturity, documented in child studies, is a staple feature in children's literature. A key indicator of the trustworthiness and morality of characters in children's books is their willingness to take children seriously. Near the end of *The Princess and the Goblin* by George MacDonald, Curdie, who has just bravely spent time in goblin territory to uncover their vile plot, rushes to warn the guards who are protecting the princess. He is ignored because of his youth, and imprisoned. At multiple points in the story, the Princess Irene's nurse is similarly unwilling to listen to the princess about the existence of her great-grandmother, something that confuses the princess and undermines her own faith in the presence of the wise woman. There are myriad other examples, like Elliot Taylor's family's disbelief about the existence of E. T. in Steven Spielberg's classic 1982 film, or Elizabeth Clarry's persistent inability in Jaclyn Moriarty's *Feeling Sorry for Celia* to get her father to attend to anything she says, including her dislike of wine. In my own childhood, the experiences of these characters resonated with my own experiences of being disbelieved, though I was never so lucky as to meet an alien.

This dismissal of children as being too immature or simply unable to express their viewpoints is tied to particular beliefs about language and the capacities necessary for truthful expression. Many people hold that meaningful communication requires a certain model of rational cognition. Extreme forms of this viewpoint insist that a proposition is only meaningful if it is verifiable. We encountered one example of how this perspective operates in our culture in the previous chapter: There is an enduring belief that for children to meaningfully communicate about death, they need to understand what death is—and children, lacking the capacity for an abstract grasp of the concept of death, cannot possibly understand it. However, when researchers talked to children directly, they discovered that, in fact, children as young as four or five had quite sophisticated understandings of death and dying.

This realization, that children understand and grieve death, has led to slow but important changes in how we respond to and care for children in the face of death.

Assessments of children's ability to communicate are biased by latent cultural assumptions about what constitutes real knowledge and expression. As Susan Wright explains in relation to children's authoring in arts-based research,

> [There is a] social and cultural dominance of *literal* language and *written* modes of expression. Such beliefs and curricular practices may be related to the underlying assumption that if something is not expressed through spoken or written language, it is considered to be outside rational thought, outside articulate feeling. Yet language as a communicational medium is inadequate for the expression of everything that we think, feel or sense.[2]

There is a tendency in Western culture to be skeptical of information that is gained through play or narrative; that is, through symbol, rather than through literal language and abstract formulation—as if these are two divergent forms of symbolization. As I described in the first chapter, this general cultural distrust has its roots in the suspicion of primitive, mythical forms of knowing and overvaluation of rational, positivist epistemologies. But because children communicate primarily through creative and artistic means, this distrust specifically invalidates children's ability to accurately relay their experiences.

Alongside its preoccupation with children's limited capacity for using literal, and especially written, modes of language, our culture also gives significant weight to children's supposed inability to distinguish real from unreal, as exemplified in their belief in certain mythical cultural beings such as Santa Claus and the Tooth Fairy. Piaget, for example, held that the ability to make basic ontological distinctions was not in place before age twelve, while more recent research has shown this basic ability in children as young as three. Nevertheless, children's proclivity to believe in fantastical beings continues to garner attention.[3]

I cannot help but wonder if these assumptions about the unreliability of children's communication partly explain the paucity of research into children's experiences in the hospital system more generally, including the lack of research into children's experiences of dying. They are certainly not the entire reason; as I noted last chapter, a key factor is the impetus to protect children from unnecessary burdens that supposedly deliver no clear benefit (unlike, apparently, drug trials). Moreover, those who do conduct this type of research into children's experiences often note that they are working against cultural and institutional beliefs. Many people, including some who work in pediatric care, don't realize just how recent these initiatives are. Since the 1950s, only a small cohort within medical research has focused on the particular experiences of children in medical contexts.[4] Communicating directly with children about their experiences has been the exception, not the rule; as recently as the 1970s and 1980s, children were routinely not assessed for pain.[5] It is quite possible that general notions about the unreliability of children's communication shape both the general medical culture as well as the surrounding society.

But regardless of to what extent assumptions about children's unreliable communication is a factor in our priorities and attitudes toward medical research, it is unquestionably the case that this view of children affects their communication within the medical environment. As Imelda Coyne puts it, "Hospitalised children are at risk of having their rights overlooked or disregarded due to the perception that they are immature and/or that they are incapable of expressing their views and opinions."[6] One excellent example of this is Nova et al.'s discourse analysis of conversations between parents, physicians, and children in a clinic environment. These researchers analyzed the contributions children made to the conversations, as well as the adult responses. They found that despite the fact that the children, aged two to six, did not speak much during these interactions, they were actively engaged and their communication was on topic. That is, the children were communicating about aspects of their experiences, either of being sick or of being in the doctor's office. However, a second finding was that despite the relevance of the children's interjections, the parents and physicians often disregarded the substantive meaning of what the children were attempting to communicate or disregarded the contributions entirely. Few of the interactions met what the researchers describe as "integration," in which the "child's contributions get accepted and elaborated by the adults, both on a content and a relational level."[7] The children's contributions were frequently discounted as being not meaningful with respect to their content and not indicative of the children's interest in the proceedings.

In one described interaction, the physician reprimanded a mother for not following the antibiotic protocol properly. The child of six interjected with her own interpretation of what medication does and, by implication, why it was necessary to use it properly. The physician responded by calling the child a "wily one," shifting the meaning of the interaction from the content level to the relational. In another, the physician responded on a semantic level to a child's question of "What?" regarding a medication, by repeating the name of the medication, but failed to understand the child's meaning, which was an inquiry about what the medication was for. Frequently, the adults codified the child's interjections as an emotional response (it makes him happy, afraid, etc.) and returned this interpretation to the child (you are afraid) without paying attention to the child's meaning. In several examples, the child's interjection was dismissed completely, or rejected as incorrect, as in the case of a child who corrected her mother on when her scabs appeared. The mother rejected the information, and the physician did not follow up in any way.

Nova's findings reflect and articulate a recent realization in pediatric literature that finds insufficient space is given to children's expressions of their own experiences of illness and active interest in the clinic environment and their own medical care.[8] As the authors of the study go on to explain, this is troubling not only because it is disrespectful to child patients, but because behavior in institutional spaces is socialized. Parents and physicians are, whether they realize it or not, training a child in how they should behave in the clinical setting. Thus, several encounters where their voices are disregarded "could favour an internal representation of the visit as a place where one should be passive and does not get heard or understood."[9] In the case of children with life-limiting illness, it is possible that the silencing effects of the socialization that goes on in medical interactions persist even as the child ends up in specific pediatric inpatient settings where more attention is given to their assertions.

The dominance of literal modes of communication is reinforced in the norms and cultures of the medical system. The hospital is a place where utilitarian categories reign supreme, from the policies and procedures regarding medical care to the principlist moral system governing medical ethics. Policies and procedures are important, but they can also lead to a separation between the physician and patient, a fixation on what is correct rather than the individual needs of a particular person, especially when that person is deemed incapable or immature. Recall Margaret Mohrmann's story of her irritation with a teenage patient who kept chasing her down because of inadequate pain control. Mohrmann, a young physician at the time, was more willing to trust the dosage listings than to listen to the experience of her patient. It was not until Mohrmann believed the teenager when she said her pain control was inadequate and engaged the patient in dialogue about her pain control that they were able to find a solution.[10]

Being heard and listened to is extremely important to children. In general, children desire to participate in their own medical care, though the extent to which this is true varies, of course, on a case-by-case basis.[11] This is in part because, as in Mohrmann's story, this is necessary for adequate treatment. Children want to be well informed about procedures and treatments; effective communication with children is correlated with lower levels of pain and anxiety. Even though children report becoming accustomed to being passive in medical interactions, this still causes them frustration and distress.[12] In these medical studies, and in the myriad interactions we have with children in day-to-day life, it is clear that children *themselves* view their communication as meaningful and important too. They have views and opinions about their own experiences, about the hospital system, about their bodies, and about their social context that they are eager to share.

As befits the intentions of this book, I do not intend to offer practical, clinical guidelines for communication with children. I leave that to the experts. Instead, in this chapter I will explore children's communication by explicating a theory of language in which language is bound up in experience, and for which the capacity for language already assumes meaningful communication. In other words, in order to listen to children and to research their experiences, we must see that children *can* meaningfully express their experiences. To see *how* this is the case, I will consider what we think experiences are, how they can be expressed, and how they are related to judgments of fact and judgments of value. Experience is not limited to certain bodily sensations or to emotions, but encompasses the whole person: bodily, emotional, communal, aesthetic, intellectual. The meaning of any idea or concept is not explicit and fixed, already out there in the world. It is not hidden in our experiences, waiting for language to display it accurately.

Instead, the meaningfulness of a child's experience is generated in their attempts to symbolize it, both to themselves and to others. These attempts often take creative means—art or play—and are brought to fruition in back-and-forth communication with others in which the experiences are further symbolized and interpreted. Imagination and art are ways in which children transform themselves and the world around them. They not only inherit meanings, but play with them, make new meanings, and communicate these meanings to others. Because meaning can be shared and communicated in all these various ways, meaning-making allows for a collaboration, where the search for knowledge can be undertaken together.

It is important to remember that children's communication about their experiences and their views is not simply an expression of their thoughts in the abstract, regardless of context. Children's expressions arise *within conversation and in response to others around them.* Their speech is wrapped up in a shared endeavor to understand, and not simply a contextless expression of their interior thoughts and experience. It is communication between persons and, as such, meaningful.[13] Within the medical context, children's expressions of meaning are directed at their parents, health-care professionals, friends, and siblings—that is, toward those around them. But of course, just because a child's communication is meaningful does not mean it represents a fully developed judgment of fact or value. In this chapter, then, I will talk about how this shared communication can happen across levels of meaning.

While I do not hold to theories of language that require a certain level of rational capacity in order for meaningful communication, it is nonetheless true that children's ability to effectively communicate their experiences in relation to a particular concrete reality is intimately related to the communication that they receive. This is because children's manner of communicating often differs from that of adolescents and adults in significant ways. It tends to be less formal, and to involve fantasy, play, and art. Thus, we need to consider the constraints of medical (and other cultural) institutions in children's communication, both the constraints these institutions place on children's communication, and the constraints that the institutional systems place on those who work in them. As I will discuss more in the following chapter, even settings where children's communication is recognized are largely in institutional contexts driven by adult goals and modes of communication.[14] Even though it is generally recognized that children have the right to participate in their own medical care, the arrangements of space and time in the hospital are rarely conducive to sustained interaction, even if children are included in conversations or if communication is spontaneously instigated by the child.[15] Research shows that many children do not consider the explanations they receive from physicians to be communicated at a level appropriate for their understanding. This is in contrast with physicians; in one study, 90 percent of them considered their communication to be at an appropriate level.[16]

Children require support from the other active members of the conversation to enrich their semantic and relational meaning.[17] The fact that children can meaningfully communicate does not mean it is easy for us to understand or research them. It also means that their meaningful communication, as it arises in interactions with others, is significantly affected by whether there is what linguists call integration, as described above. Child researchers report that there are many more opportunities for taking a child's perspective if researchers properly adapt methods to facilitate children's participation.[18] But even if there is increasing acceptance that children are able to express their views and should be included in decision-making, putting this into practice is still largely dependent on factors such as parental buy-in, structural support, and access to high-quality pediatric care (children's hospitals will be much better set up to include children, and much likelier to have the resources and specialists to facilitate this).

But as active members in the conversation, who often communicate in creative and fantastical ways, children also model communicative alternatives to adults. Thus, we should see children's communication not only in terms of immaturity and incompleteness, though of course this is, in part, true. What child grasps the intricacies of open-heart surgery? At the same time, children remind us that the cultural dominance of literal and written modes of communication are insufficient for many of our communicative needs, especially when it comes to making meaning in difficult circumstances. In the same way that children are genuine moral agents even though they are not full, responsible moral agents (whatever that means, and if any of us meet that criteria), children communicate meaningfully. In the same way that children have something to teach us about the moral life, children have something to teach us about how to communicate.

✳✳✳

Throughout the medical studies I have cited in the first section of this chapter, two interrelated concepts appear again and again: the ability of children to *meaningfully* and *accurately* express their thoughts and feelings about themselves, with a focus here on the medical context.[19] These terms, and the relationship between them, are rarely defined, though they are generally used interchangeably. To what end do we ask children about their level of pain, the cause of their accident, their preferences regarding room setup and hospital design, or whether the intervention has made them feel better, if they cannot be trusted to answer accurately? Similarly, if children have undeveloped understandings of death, of the future consequences and implications of various treatment options, and of their preferred place to die, then it does not make sense to ask their opinions on such meaningful matters. Concerns about accuracy are often undergirded with the assumption that children have too poor a recall, and that they are too influenced by suggestion, thus rendering us unsure as to whether what they express is truly "their own" or something suggested to them.[20] This last issue, that of undue influence, is important, but only if it is raised in the context of an understanding of how meanings are symbolized, and of the dialogical nature of symbolization.[21]

To start with concerns about accuracy is to get off on the wrong foot. To ask whether an expression or symbolization—in verbal or nonverbal form—is "true" or "accurate" is the wrong question, because it assumes a language behind language, a realm of pure experience that language must then bridge. I say a language behind a language because that "pure experience" must itself exist in some way that can be understood or expressed, some internal or latent symbolization that we must feel matches our external or explicit symbolization or conceptual definition. Since children lack abstract language capacities that would allow them to make this bridge, their ability to accurately express an experience is often doubted. But asking whether the expression is accurate in this way misunderstands how meaning is created and how concepts function. The mediation that occurs is not between some sort of "experiential meaning unit" trapped inside the child needing accurate symbolization and the wider world. The more relevant question is whether children's expressions *mean* their experience, or whether their expressions are detached from or adjacent to their experiencing.

Charles Taylor calls this theory of a language behind a language *enframing theory*.[22] Cartesian in its theoretical underpinnings, it presupposes an external reality and a set of internal ideas. Accurate knowledge requires that the internal ideas match up with the external reality. Words aid the association between the ideas and the reality; they are effective signs whose correctness lies in whether they match description with object. Significantly, the internal ideas and external reality (that is, how a human being functions mentally in the world) exist mostly or entirely independent of language. Language is supremely useful, but not necessary. In this theory, children begin with animal-like natural signs, that is, noises, connected to an idea. As they develop language, they replace that sign with a more sophisticated sign, a word, which allows them to focus on a particular idea and to manipulate it. Words are a way of controlling reality.

Think, for example, of the way a young child uses the term "yesterday" to describe the past in an undifferentiated way. "I went to the zoo yesterday," she might say, when in fact it was three months ago, or "Grandma and Grandpa came to our house yesterday," when in fact it was last year. In this case, according to enframing theory, we say that her use of the term is wrong, because it does not match up correctly to what yesterday actually is. Thus, the child's statement that "I went to the zoo yesterday" is inaccurate, predicated on an insufficient mental idea—that is, an immature and incomplete grasp of the abstract concept of time.

A contrasting approach is what Taylor calls the *constitutive* model of language. Here I find the work of Eugene Gendlin and Bernard Lonergan most helpful in expressing the implications of this model for the relationship between language and experience, not least because it ties into the account of cognitive and ethical intentionality I described in the first two chapters of this book. In this theory, the meaning-content of any idea or word is not explicit and fixed, already out there in the world. It is not hidden in our experiences, waiting for language to display it accurately. That is, this theory explicitly rejects the idea that the world and the human being in it are made up of external reality and internal ideas. Instead, "meaning is formed in the interaction of experiencing and something that functions symbolically." Gendlin calls this interaction "felt meaning."[23] For Gendlin,

> Experience is a constant, ever-present, underlying phenomenon of inwardly sentient living, and therefore there is an experiential side of anything, no matter how specifically detailed and finely specified, no matter whether it is a concept, an observed act, an inwardly felt behavior, or a sense of a situation.[24]

In other words, even the most abstract and theoretical concepts are grounded in felt meaning that exists, not out there in the world, but in persons.

If you cast your mind back to chapter 2, I briefly explained Lonergan's four levels of consciousness. This ever-present reality, experience, is one of the four levels of conscious intentionality (together with understanding, reason, and judgment), and indispensable for human knowing. The level of experience consists in empirical operations, those of sensing, perceiving, imagining, feeling, speaking, and moving. What a child (or anyone) experiences, she then comes to understand.[25] This is the process of further symbolization. Experience is not something that simply happens to a child, as it were, but yields a mode of intending, where her senses attend to her self and the world around her. That is, her experience is patterned. She—and children are not unique here—does not experience a pure external reality, as is imagined in the enframing theory. Her very experience is formed in the process of symbolization.

By patterned, I mean that the attentiveness of her experience is selective due to the fact that experience does not exist independently from intentional consciousness, nor from symbolization, but rather experience, understanding, reasoning, and judgment are integrated in the unity of consciousness; in our practice of knowing, we experience them as a unity and only differentiate them upon reflection. So, we do not experience only, but what we experience is patterned by what we understand, know, and do. How we notice, understand, and characterize our experiences is determined by the meanings we have inherited and created, such that there is no pure experience that comes before any meanings. These experiences can then be symbolized and interpreted "further and further" to the extent that "[they] can be differentiated and symbolized in the formation of very many meanings."[26] There is thus no simple correspondence between idea and reality that can be expressed in the correct word. Instead, there are a variety of constitutive symbolizations.

But it would be a mistake to think of a child's experience here as a merely bodily (animal-like) one that will be grasped by her developing cognitive abilities. Experience is not limited to mere bodily patterns. In addition to the biological pattern of experience, Lonergan describes aesthetic and intellectual patterns. The aesthetic pattern of experience is joyful and breaks the bonds of the biological drive—it is the realm of the spontaneous, the flexible, the fantastical. There is also the intellectual pattern of experience, where consciousness is dominated by the desire to know, to formulate logically what is experienced in other ways.[27] Thus, *this account of the creation of meaning does not exclude the logical orders.* Experience and logic are linked because experience, as Gendlin puts it, "functions in the *formation* of meaning and logical orders."[28] Human experience, when objectified by the philosopher, can be separated into these different patterns of experience in this manner, but in everyday living, there is no differentiation between them. Instead, there is a flow of patterned experience, where one may move between patterns without noticing. Experiencing is the "flow of feeling, concretely, to which you can every moment attend inwardly, if you wish."[29] Thus, experience is not limited to certain bodily sensations or to emotions, but encompasses the whole person: bodily, emotional, communal, aesthetic, and intellectual.

The meaningfulness of a child's experience is generated in their attempts to symbolize it, both to themselves and to others, and is further symbolized and interpreted in communication with others. This is how children learn and develop, according to Lev Vygotsky. Instead of seeing development, as Piaget does, as preceding learning—that is, seeing the development of capacities for knowledge as the "unfolding of some genetic or neurological imperative"—Vygotsky describes the acquisition of knowledge capacity as a primarily social endeavor.[30] Learning unfolds through social collaboration, through the dialogical process between the child and others, whether they are more advanced peers or adults. Key to Vygotsky's idea is the gulf that grows continually wider between what a child can do on her own, and what a child can do through this back-and-forth with others. This type of learning can be seen in adult interactions as well; Gendlin describes this process of creation of meaning in the adult therapeutic relationship.[31]

Thus, experience and meaning are intimately related. Experiencing subjects live in a world mediated by meaning, where meaning is not abstracted from the subject, but rather arises from the subject and is shared communally. "Meaning is an act that does not merely repeat but goes beyond experiencing."[32] It goes beyond but cannot be separated from experiencing specifically because meaning is found in the interaction between experience and symbolization. Meaning is communicated in many ways: "intersubjectively, artistically, symbolically, linguistically, incarnately."[33] Meaning can be expressed; in turn, the hearer or reader may respond, and this expression and response need not be on the same level, but could be words in response to a picture, for example. This is the back-and-forth in which symbolization is refined and further meanings created. This communication of meaning leads to the creation of generalized concepts, to communal meaning, and it is the communal that makes knowledge possible: We are dependent on others for the meaning and values by which we live.[34]

When children first learn language, they learn not only words but meanings—they learn verbal symbols to explicate the felt meaning of their experiences, symbols that also shape those experiences. Language is not grounded, then, in some external reality with which the child must align her mental image and her vocabulary. Instead, language is grounded in the felt meaning of the child as a knowing subject. The fact that children are inter-subjective and self-transcending subjects, as I argued in the first two chapters, has ramifications too for how we think about their communication. Children do not live in their own intellectual realm but already engage in the same operations, and the same levels of intentional consciousness, as adults. Because of this, infants and children can share with their older peers and with adults a joint attention to an object which is then symbolized, usually by a word. When a parent says "come here" and waves a child over, the child perceives the communicative intent and learns the words for that intent. Inasmuch as children are constituted by others, and humans are constituted by language, children are inherently meaningful communicators.

So, to return to the child's use of "yesterday." A young child will often also refer to "a long, long time ago," for example, "A long, long, long time ago when I was a baby . . ." Objectively, perhaps, it was not such a long time ago. But the use of "yesterday" and "a long, long time ago" depict the child's knowledge that things have happened in the near and far past. Furthermore, it is possible that things that happened "yesterday" are things that feel recent to the child, as opposed to things that happened "a long, long, long time ago." This is meaningful and accurate to their feelings, even though it does not map perfectly onto the differentiated language used by adults who have a tendency to think in calendar terms. When we tell a child "You were a baby a long time ago," we are not giving them words to depict some objective reality, but shaping those experiences. Crucial here is the concept that the child learns these felt meanings in the embodied experience of time connected with words, rather than in an abstract grasp of the concept of time as such.

✳✳✳

Let us return to the question that drives this chapter: Does a child mean what she says? In the previous section, I rejected the idea that meaningful commu-nication depends on a particular model of rational cognition. Instead, what a child says arises from her felt meaning. The meaningfulness of her experience then takes shape in her attempts to symbolize it using symbolizations that are largely given to her by others. Now I turn to the topic of how children communicate, and how we should think about their communicative acts.

Even if children are not too immature for meaningful communication, it is important to recognize that their grasp of language and abstract concepts, and their ability to express their thoughts in literal, verbal, and written forms, are underdeveloped. Thus, when we ask "does a child mean what she says?" we should be aware of how we expect her to "say" it.

Children communicate meaning. But in what ways? They do communicate in statements of fact: "I want the blue hat; I do not want crust on my sandwiches; I do not need to go to bed because I am not tired." And most of these, with the exception of the last one, have a high chance of being true to a child's experience. While significant attention has been given to children's fantasy, much daily communication with even very young children involves statements of fact. Children are often eager to verbally report what happened at daycare or school, what is new in their friends' lives, or what they have learned about fire safety. Children also intentionally play with truth and falsehood in their statements of fact, as when a child points to a cat and says "This is a dog!" amid peals of laughter. Through their words, children play with symbolizations to wake new meanings.

But both in and out of the medical context, children primarily symbolize their experiences and communicate complex ideas through a mixture of literal language, play, art, and stories:

> Hence, drawing, graphic-narrative play and other forms of artistic expression offer important and distinct forms of meaning-making through figurative communication, which is intricate, multifaceted, symbolic and metaphoric. . . . Such open-ended, personal forms of knowing, expressing and communicating unleash and reveal children's deep meaning, multiple perspective-taking and fluidity of thought.[35]

Sometimes this artistic and playful communication is explicit communication of a given idea or event, as when a child draws a picture and interprets it. The need for interpretation is often a surprise to the child; it is generally so obvious to the child what the drawing is that they are frustrated by the inability of adults to immediately apprehend their meaning. One can remember here the surprise of the Little Prince in Antoine de Saint-Exupéry's story at the inability of the adults around him to understand his drawing of the elephant who was eaten by the snake. To children, the symbolization is perfectly adequate as an expression of their felt meaning.

There are also less explicit ways of communicating through art, play, or stories. For example, sometimes a child needs to reenact an event over and over again, or desires to hear the same story multiple times. In play therapy, children will often reenact the same event repeatedly.[36] Izetta Smith tells the story of a three-year-old whose sister died in a mountain accident playing the event over and over, pulling on someone's arm in an imitation of the rescue effort. Finally, other children came to help her, and pulled together. The children ended up falling on the floor together in laughter. In another example, Loretta M. Kopelman and John C. Moskop describe the popularity of *Charlotte's Web* among children who are dying, who want to hear over and over again the passages about Charlotte's death.[37] Rather than making direct statements about their dying, these children express their knowledge of their prognoses through demanding the story. In Myra Bluebond-Langner's study of dying children, she found that children often communicated their knowledge that they were dying through play, as in the example of one girl who made paper dolls and would bury them in Kleenex boxes.[38]

As knowing persons, children are experiencing subjects who live in a world mediated by meaning. They engage with the world through their imagination. Contrary to accounts that are "in line with the notion of the small child as a creature living in a world of dreams, hazy impressions, and symbols," and see imagination as a flight of fancy which serves no purpose and disregards reality, I follow thinkers who see the imagination as realistic and necessary to knowledge.[39] Imagination allows children, adolescents, and adults to play with a multiplicity of meaning through the selection of further symbolization, and lets us open up new ways to understand reality. This is why medieval theologians often described imagination as the handmaid of reason; it is what allows the contemplative to go from that which is visible to that which is invisible. It is the imagination that allows us to move easily between "the general and the particular; the necessary and the random; the notional and the real; the known and the unknown."[40] Imagination is not separate from the reality of a child, but rather "a child's experience of life is filtered through the imagination . . . and fact and fantasy may be inextricably linked in how a child represents a real life experience."[41]

This linking of the two is not contrary to but necessary for "real" knowing, and crucial in how children express their experiences and viewpoints, and how they make meaning for themselves. Children use imagination to create meaning to understand both themselves and the world around them. Thus, when Taylor says that "language cannot be generated from within; it can only come to the child from her milieu—although once it is mastered, innovation becomes possible," he misses the point.[42] Long before children master language, in the sense that they grasp a significant range of vocabulary and grammatical and syntactical conventions, children innovate all the time through metaphor, multivalent meaning, and even nonsense, as in the case of Diamond in MacDonald's story.

In fact, children have an amazing ability to make meaning where we may have thought that it was impossible. Children constantly engage in creative patterning and reorganization of their experience through different symbolizations, presenting new insights when the old insights are just not helping. An example of this can be seen in a research-intervention project for children with cancer between the ages of six and ten, in which the children invented fairy tales.[43] Researchers found in this fairy tale storytelling multiple levels of meaning. Through telling stories about the experiences and actions of the characters, the children also explored and communicated various aspects of their own experiences, such as feelings of pain or isolation. For example, the tales gave meaning to suffering. The children played, through the characters, with ideas of companionship and mutual support. And through the stories, they connected with larger ideas of good versus evil. Through this multivalency of meaning, the children were able to make meaning of their own situation indirectly, rather than through simple factual statements. But they did not only make meaning; through storytelling, the children *shaped* their experience of illness. This illustrates my point that the meaningfulness of a child's experiences is shaped through symbolization. As Margherita, et al. write, "The fantasy has constructed meanings about the illness, hospital, relatives and doctors, etc. providing a new solution to the conflicts."[44]

Children can also use creative and metaphorical meanings to express their understanding of disease. In a paper on children's perceptions of asthma, Jane Peterson and Yvonne Sterling explore the ways in which children use metaphors to make sense of the disease, as well as to understand themselves and their own emotions in relation to it.[45] In their study, they list various ways children use metaphors to think about their asthma: as a bubble, as a constant companion, as an intruder, as an unpredictable visitor, as a troll, as crackers, as a guardian angel, and as a jellyfish. The way in which these children understand their asthma is an example of metaphorical language, where the lived experiences of these children are transferred to unconventional but interpretable linguistic forms. Importantly, these unconventional forms demonstrate a good understanding of asthma, and give the children a sense of agency in managing their illness. In the variety of metaphors used, each depicts triggers, airway responsiveness and limitation, and associated symptoms. For many of the children in Peterson and Sterling's study, there is a direct link between their chosen image(s), and the warning signs that their asthma has been triggered—that is, these metaphorical understandings help children to be participants in their own care. Before the harsh stings of a jellyfish, explains one of the children, there is a gentle brushing up of tentacles, warning the child to change course.

Lonergan's and Gendlin's ideas about the art and artistic patterns of experience help to organize and differentiate the behaviors mentioned above and validate them as integral to a child's developing reasonable subjectivity. Artistic symbolization is not an inferior form of symbolization. The statement that these are "personal forms of knowledge" is not a denigration when we realize that all forms of knowledge are ultimately personal and that language is grounded in a subject's felt meaning. The symbolizations that play a role in the creation of meaning include not just theoretical linguistic symbols, but also nontheoretical linguistic symbols, and nonlinguistic symbolization.[46] These nonverbal symbols are crucial to knowledge. As Lonergan puts it, "The aesthetic liberation and the free artistic control of the flow of sensations and images, of emotions and bodily movements, do not merely break the bonds of biological drive but also generate in experience a flexibility that makes it a ready tool for the spirit of inquiry."[47] In shying away from metaphor and other forms of imagistic language, we not only implicitly discourage children from interpreting their own subjective experiences through particular narrative forms, but we miss the possibilities of metaphorical rupture that children effect, where they change themselves, others, and their situation through the creative inbreaking of new meaning.

This need of children to use art and imagination to express their experiences should not surprise us. In fact, it reminds us that it is a very real need for adults too, as music, art, and poetry convey emotion and experiences in a way that is different from and deeper than simple statements of fact. To put this in Lonerganian terms, children have something to teach us. "For teaching is the communication of insight. It throws out clues, the pointed hints, that lead to insight. . . . It pits the further questions that reveal the need of further insights to modify and complement the acquired store."[48] In a dialogue, the supplier of insight and the poser of further questions need not be the same person. And this is where we can clearly see the way that children have something to teach us. They often ask further questions, through imagination and creative leaps, that do not occur to adults. They have spontaneous insights. While they lack the store of knowledge that an adult possesses, they are also less constrained by repeated patterns. They "provoke the contradictions that direct . . . attention to what [has been] overlooked."[49] Children, in their capacity for meaning-making, can provoke us to a deeper understanding of them, ourselves, and the world.

Because meaning can be shared and communicated in all these ways, meaning-making allows for a collaborative approach, where the search for knowledge can be (must be?) undertaken together. Children and their more advanced peers or adults do not need to engage in the same acts of meaning or at the same level of expression; they need not be intellectual equals. They can engage in a back-and-forth of further symbolization in which the symbols do not need to be identical, or even of the same kind.[50] A potential act of meaning made by a child may still be communicated to a parent or peer, who can help with or complete the task of thinking, formulating, and judging. Similarly, a parent or health-care professional can help a child come to a judgment regarding the truth of what they understand about their experience. In play therapy, for example, meaning is expressed by a child through bodily movement and artistic creations, and then formulated into an abstract notion by the therapist. Both thus learn what the child is experiencing and help meet the needs of the child in that experience. When adults and advanced peers express and reflect to children an appreciation of their felt meanings, the child is invited to refine their sense of these meanings in and to themselves. This refining can even help to recharacterize an experience: Felt meaning can be changed in the process of comprehension.[51] We sometimes see that we did not really understand something until we tried to express it.

Through this collaborative approach, children are able to accomplish more than they could alone. This is why researchers found dramatically different results in children's understandings of death from studies of healthy children when they interviewed children who were ill and in hospital settings.[52] It was primarily a lack of experience and collaborative symbolization, rather than a lack of fixed biological capacity for cognition, that interfered with children's understanding of death. All of the children Bluebond-Langner studied came to understand themselves, their disease trajectory, and their impending death in similar ways, despite significant age variation. In her study, children as young as five came to the same understanding as children of ten.[53] I do not want to be misunderstood here—I am not suggesting that children do not have significant limitations based on their age or stage of development. Children are incapable of understanding certain things; for example, it is hard to imagine any kind of appropriate way to communicate the intricacies of open-heart surgery and its many potential outcomes weighed against nonsurgical interventions to a four-year-old. However, we should not be too prescriptive about what children can and cannot understand based on a "cognitively" determined scale, which views the child as an individual removed from context.

This model of communication has implications for how we judge children's capacity to participate in medical conversations.[54] We should think of capacity not in general, nor even for this or that particular decision, which is how capacity is generally defined in hospitals. Instead, assessments of capacity should take into account the communicative context of the child, health-care professionals, and family, and the extent to which the child can acquire the necessary cognitive and emotional skills in collaboration with others. I'll return to this idea in the next chapter.

A collaborative approach also means that a child's environment will significantly shape her experience. When we see that language arises communally, and that children receive language from others, we should be attentive to the ways in which language can shape children's experiences and understanding in harmful ways. For example, because actions, routines, and bodily patterns are also communicative, children often feel guilty about their illness and think that it is a punishment.[55] This is in part because the necessities of treatment—like having to stay in their room or not being able to go to a party—mimic punishments for bad behavior.

In the introduction to this chapter, I discussed the concern of some researchers that children's lack of integration in clinical settings trains them for passivity in those settings. But our language and symbolizations do not simply train children in expected behavior; what we tell children about their bodies and their disease shapes their experience of those things. For example, consider the popularity of battle imagery and military metaphors in pediatric medicine (and medicine in general). These images position children as metaphorical soldiers, both vocally—"he's such a brave little soldier" or "she's a fighter"—and through larger public narratives, like the SickKids Toronto ad campaign, whose triumphalist imagery includes children in military costumes.[56] This framework can shape the experience of children, compounding the silencing of children that already occurs in medical settings. Children, like soldiers, are never in command. An ideal soldier is obedient, brave, self-sacrificial, and does not question their commanding officers. The ideal soldier does not exercise his or her individual decision-making agency but conforms. This image thus reinforces the cultural structures of obedience in the role of child. Military imagery also does little to create forms of meaning that help children learn to be at peace with their bodies. It has little to offer children with chronic illness and is especially troubling in its implications for children who die, who lose the fight.

On the other hand, while it is unfortunate that our cultural emblems of strength are almost always violent, there is no guarantee that when a child invokes military imagery, they mean the same things we mean. If children are drawing on their own subjective lived histories whereby they have learned about imagery, characters, and plot, they may not be thinking about modern warfare with the virtues and issues listed above. They may instead be imagining St. George fighting the dragon, or the Pevensie children fighting the White Witch's animal hordes. In the fairy tale storytelling group, the fictional use of conflict became a narrative way to overcome conflicts in the child's life. What is important is that we understand the way in which story, imagery, and metaphor shape experience, and from that foundation engage with children in their adoption of these storylines, being aware of the ways in which they may be interactionally compelled to conform to a given image or cultural expectation.

The ability to use symbolization to shape children's experiences often has an unclear overlap with the stories that children create about their own situations. Jane Peterson argues that children's metaphors should be respected as meaningful, but she does not discuss potentially troubling metaphorical language use. For example, one of the children in the study imagines her asthma as a guardian angel whose presence means that the child no longer needs her medicine. In the child's words, "The guardian angel sent by God helps me to be good. However, if I mess up, I will get into trouble. My guardian angel does not protect me and can even take the air away."

This is an example of the "adoption of a storyline which incorporates a particular interpretation of cultural stereotypes to which interlocutors are interactionally compelled to conform."[57] Respect for a child's language and other expressions of her experience does not mean that we ought to leave them unquestioned or unchallenged. Instead, they are part of a shared dialogue. In this case, a key question that comes to mind is where the child may have gotten this idea. Let us not forget that, rightly intentioned or not, parents often lie to their children to ensure their protection or obedience. So it is possible she heard this from her parents. But it is equally possible that she drew this connection for herself. Does that make it less problematic? In some ways, yes. But in terms of our responsibilities to help children nurture good relationships with themselves, no. "Outside influence" is not inherently a problem—in acts of shared language, where metaphors are co-constructed, it is not an aberration but the only way things can be communicated and created. But we should be cautious about undue influence in communication, about what storylines children have in mind, about how these ideas affect their relationships, their sense of self, and their understanding of illness.

Jane Peterson rightly advocates for the use of metaphor in the interaction between children and health-care professionals, but she overestimates the difference between clinical language and metaphorical language, as if clinical language is devoid of metaphor, and metaphor is the opposite of literal language. Metaphoric language is not language whose meaning diverges from its truer or more literal semantic denotation, but language by which the lived experiences of social actors are transferred to unconventional but interpretable linguistic forms.[58] She also leaves largely unexplored the ways in which metaphorical language is established locally in interaction and co-constructed. Her underdevelopment of the relationship between the clinical language of the health-care providers and the metaphorical language used by children reflects a more general lack of research on the relationship between metaphorical frameworks used in clinical settings and children's experiences of their disease.

Earlier in this chapter, I said that it is wrong to think of children's expressions of their experience as mediation between some experiential meaning unit trapped inside the child and accurate symbolization. In the pediatric medical context, there is instead mediation between the spontaneous symbolizations of the child (including nonverbal symbols) and the linguistic systems of symbolization of medical and ethical reasoning. Children are not a unique case here; this mediation occurs for all of us, though there is of course a difference between children's and adults' experiences of it. Medical and ethical discourse properly has its own type of symbolizations in which theoretical linguistic symbols play a crucial role. This discourse relies heavily on general-ized concepts, such that we often fail to see that these definitional elements of these concepts are also symbols, and those in turn can function as definitions specifically because they are grounded in felt meaning.[59] This is no separate realm of knowledge, for all its technical jargon. Linguistic symbolization is but one possible form of symbolization that expresses our experience and is only better when and insofar as it is a more effective symbolization of the experience. Logical elements necessary for ethical discourse are not detached from subjective meaning, from experience, because if they were, they would have no content. Medicine and ethics too rely on felt meanings.

Thus, even if you accept that children cannot participate in the mode of reasoning that powers formally ethical or medical discourse, it does not follow that children cannot participate at all in the processes this discourse articulates, nor that they are too immature to make their experiences and opinions known in the medical setting. Children's ability to participate and communicate is becoming more and more recognized, and increasingly codified in laws and declarations of rights in many jurisdictions. But these changes do not always translate to clinical practice. Here, then, we lose the opportunities to integrate children's understandings into our own and help them develop on a content and relational level. We miss the possibilities for enriching collaboration. In back-and-forth communication that welcomes the symbolization of the child's experiences, our own understandings of the situation and of our and the child's values are constantly challenged and refined. Excluding children's own versions of their experiences and understanding makes it unlikely that we will ask and answer all relevant questions about a child's medical experience and any related decisions. Providing proper medical care to children requires that we include them.

***

Can a child mean what she says? Yes! But what a child says also shapes what she means, in the endless symbolization that shapes her experiences. Children are not simply passive recipients of knowledge; they work to both make meaning of their experiences and express meaning through a variety of symbolizations, including statements of fact, metaphor, play, art, imagination, and fantasy. They do this in collaboration with others, where further symbolization is a creative exchange between intersubjective and knowing subjects. Literal and fantastical-metaphorical languages are not opposed to each other but are both grounded in felt meaning and represent symbolizations through which experience is made meaningful. In order to properly hear children in the medical context, we need to question prevailing theories of language and views of children's communication, especially the denigration of so-called mythical and primitive modes of communicating. We must also find child-appropriate ways of communication, both in listening and in explaining.

The knowledge children express through imagery and metaphor is real knowledge. It is not pure fantasy that stands against "real, scientific knowledge." In this way, a child's expressions of her experience should be respected. She means what she says. But this respect is not a one-way "respect of autonomy" as if the child exists independently from her surroundings and relationships (the fully formed individual unit view). Instead, the child exists in a web of relationships, and part of the responsibility of caregivers in that web is to help the child understand themselves and their circumstances through language. This help includes being willing to learn from children when their metaphorical rupture brings new meaning to established forms or reverses our cherished frameworks for making meaning out of difficult circumstances. We have a moral obligation to listen to children, to create environments where their voices and experiences are central, and where they can use unconventional but interpretable linguistic forms to create new meanings and invite new viewpoints of self and disease.

Creating these kinds of environments can dramatically shape the experience of both a child and those who are in relationship with her. One study looking at the effects of a hospital fairy garden found that not only did it provide a welcoming space for children to play and to enjoy themselves but interacting with children in the hospital fairy garden changed student nurses' perspectives on their patients. "Student nurses in this study have shifted in their thinking from a purely biomedical model of care to a more humanistic ecological model."[60] This example should be an invitation to consider the ways in which our institutional spaces, with their implicit beliefs about knowledge and personhood, shape our ability to listen to children.

Recognizing that literal language and other symbolizations do not belong to separate ways of knowing but are all symbolizations of meaning reminds us that adults also communicate in these ways and need this range of symbolization to make meaning. Thus, this understanding of children as communicative should pose questions about meaning-making and the symbolization of experience more generally. Medical research involving children generally happens in specific pediatric environments and is cut off from "normal human studies," as if children have nothing to tell us about life and medicine and the nature of experience, as if the experiences of children tell no truths about humanity at large. Instead, we need to humble ourselves and be willing to learn from children. The fact that children use the same structures of knowing and experiencing as adults means they reveal something about adults too. Childhood is not a stage of life left behind but is foundational. Creating these spaces for children benefits us too—in creating spaces for intersubjective and interpersonal connection, which we so desperately need, even if we can pretend that we don't:

> We live in a time when the fullness of these feelings [of grief] is not easily accepted or understood. We quiet our crying, our yelling is muffled or hidden away; therefore, grieving can be difficult for people who are confronted with the intensity of these feelings. They may have to learn, or relearn, how to express them. However, young children are spontaneous with their feelings. No matter what the circumstance, a child will usually cry and yell when she or he needs to, a healthy response to pain.[61]

In the same way that cities designed with children in mind tend to be the most livable for everyone, structures created for children can be helpful for everyone.[62] Health-care practitioners need to tell stories to make meaning of their experiences as much as their patients do.

We must attend to children, then, to their meaningful expressions of their experiences. Attending to children opens up the possibility that we will hear them. But because conscious intentionality is patterned, we do not perceive things equally; rather, "perceiving is a function of interest, anticipation, and activity."[63] What we experience is determined by that to which we attend. That is, our attentiveness to what children express in discourse is predicated on our expectations of the meaningfulness of what they have to say. The more we are willing to open ourselves to children, to listen to what they have to say by seeing value and validity in their communication, the better we will be able to perceive what it is they mean. We should seek to be like the good adults in children's stories, the ones who hear children and take them seriously.

As communicative subjects who mean what they say, children thus have the right to be heard and attended to in all medical interactions. We should work hard toward integration, so that children can properly collaborate with us. When I say that we need to listen to children's experiences, I mean that we need to conduct research to better understand the needs and abilities of children in the medical context, and we need to create environments in which it is the norm to have meaningful conversations characterized by respect between parents and children, between children and other children, and between children and health-care practitioners. I mean we need to change the way we view children, the veracity of their statements, the reliability of their expressions, and their own insights into themselves and their surroundings. Addressing the needs of children in the medical context means seeing value in their knowledge and ability to express their experiences. Engaging children in this way goes beyond simply addressing their immediate medical needs—though it is not less than this! Instead, seeing them as whole persons compels us to make space for their ways of being, for their development, curiosity, self-communication, play, imagination, and fantasy.

Children mean what they say. Will we listen?

NOTES

1 Nancy Scheper-Hughes, "Institutionalized Sex Abuse and the Catholic Church" in *Small Wars: The Cultural Politics of Childhood*, ed. Nancy Scheper-Hughes and Carolyn Sargent (Berkeley: University of California Press, 1998), 295–317; Sheila Ramaswamy and Shekhar Seshadri, "Our Failure to Protect Sexually Abused Children: Where is Our 'Willing Suspension of Disbelief'?" *Indian Journal of Psychiatry* 59 (2017): 233–235; UK Ministry of Justice, "Assessing Risk of Harm to Children and Parents in Private Law Children Cases Final Report," June 2020. https://tinyurl.com/378jc8m8

2 Susan Wright, "Graphic-narrative Play: Young Children's Authoring through Drawing and Telling," *International Journal of Education & the Arts* 8 (2007): 24.

3 See, for example, Jacqueline D. Woolley and Maliki Ghossainy, "Revisiting the Fantasy-Reality Distinction: Children as Naïve Skeptics," *Child Development* 84 (2013): 1496–1510.

4 See D.G. Prugh, et al., "A Study of the Emotional Reactions of Children and Families to Hospitalization and Illness," *American Journal of Orthopsychiatry* 23 (1953): 70–106; A. Rokash and M. Parvini, "Experience of Adults and Children in Hospitals," *Early Child Development and Care* 181 (2011): 707–715.

5 Elizabeth A. Ely, "The Experience of Pain for School-Age Children: Blood, Band-Aids, and Feelings," *CHC* 21 (1992): 168.

6 Imelda Coyne and Lisa Kirwan, "Ascertaining Children's Wishes and Feelings about Hospital Life," *Journal of Child Health Care* 16 (2012): 294.

7 Cristina Nova, et al., "The Physician–Patient–Parent Communication: A Qualitative Perspective on the Child's Contribution," *Patient Education and Counseling* 58 (2005): 332.

8 See Coyne and Kirwan, "Ascertaining Children's Wishes"; See also an excellent summary in Vida Jeremic, et al., "Participation of Children in Medical Decision-Making: Challenges and Potential Solutions," *Bioethical Inquiry* 13 (2016): 527.

9 Nova, et al., "Physician–Patient–Parent Communication," 332.

10 Margaret Mohrmann, *Attending Children: A Doctor's Education* (Washington, DC: Georgetown University Press, 2006), 25–26.

11 Imelda Coyne, "Consultation with Children in Hospital: Children, Parents' and Nurses' Perspectives," *Journal of Clinical Nursing* 15, (2006): 61–71.

12 Coyne and Kirwan, "Ascertaining Children's Wishes," 300; Jeremic, et al., "Participation," 525–527.

13 Erica Burman, *Deconstructing Developmental Psychology*, 3rd ed. (London: Routledge, 2017), Chapter 10. See also Nova, et al., "Physician–Patient–Parent Communication," 330.

14 Michael Wyness, "Children's Participation: Definitions, Narratives and Disputes" in *Theorising Childhood: Citizenship, Rights, and Participation*, eds. Claudio Baraldi and Tom Cockburn (London: Palgrave MacMillan, 2018), 57.

15 I. Runeson, E. Martensson, and K. Enskar, "Children's Knowledge and Degree of Participating in Decision Making when Undergoing a Clinical Diagnostic Procedure," in *Pediatric Nursing* 33 (2007): 505–511; Jeremic, et al., "Participation," 527.

16 Coyne and Kirwan, "Ascertaining Children's Wishes," 300.

17 Nova, et al., "Physician–Patient–Parent Communication," 330.

18 See Stefan Nilsson, et al., "Children's Voices—Differentiating a Child Perspective from a Child's Perspective," in *Developmental Neurorehabilitation* 18 (2015): 162–168.

19 See, among others, B. Davies, et al., "Children's Perspectives of a Pediatric Hospice Program," in *Journal of Palliative Care* 12 (2005): 253; M. D. Jerrett, "Children and Pain," in *CHC* 14 (1985): 83–89; C. S. Jensen, et al., "Children's Experiences of Acute Hospitalisation to a Paediatric Emergency and Assessment Unit—A Qualitative Study," in *Journal of Child Health Care* 16 (2012): 271; F. Bonoti, et al., "Exploring Children's Understanding of Death: Through Drawings and the Death Concept Questionnaire," in *Death Studies* 37 (2013): 48–59; C. L. von Baeyer, et al., "Can We Screen Young Children for their Ability to Provide Accurate Self-Reports of Pain?" in *Pain* 152 (2011): 1327.

20 Davies, et al., "Children's Perspectives," 253; R. Hart, Children's Participation: From Tokenism to Citizenship in *Innocenti Essays 4, UNICEF.* (Florence: Italy, 1992).

21 I follow Gendlin's expansive definition of symbolization, which includes logical, verbal definitional elements, but is not limited to these. In fact, they include all types of senses, movement, and expressions. Eugene Gendlin, *Experiencing and the Creation of Meaning: A Philosophical and Psychological Approach to the Subjective* (Evanston: Northwestern University Press, 1997), introduction.

22 See Charles Taylor, *The Language Animal: The Full Shape of the Human Linguistic Capacity* (Cambridge: Belknap Press of Harvard University Press, 2016), 3–50.

23 Gendlin, *Experiencing*, 5.

24 Gendlin, *Experiencing*, 15.

25 Bernard Lonergan, *Method in Theology* (Toronto: University of Toronto Press, 1990), 9.

26 Lonergan, *Method*, 133; Gendlin, *Experiencing*, 16; Bernard Lonergan, *Insight*, vol. 3, *The Collected Works of Bernard Lonergan* (Toronto: University of Toronto Press, 1988), 212.

27 Lonergan, *Method*, 205–211.

28 Gendlin, *Experiencing*, 3.

29 Gendlin, *Experiencing*, 3.

30 Michael K. White, *Maps of Narrative Practice* (New York: Norton, 2007), 271.

31 Gendlin, *Experiencing*, 226–274.

32 Lonergan, *Method*, 77.

33 Lonergan, *Method*, 78.

34 Lonergan, *Method*, 71–2; Gendling, *Experiencing*, 107; Bernard Lonergan, *Topics in Education*, vol. 10, *The Collected Works of Bernard Lonergan* (Toronto: University of Toronto Press, 2000), 201.

35 Wright, "Graphic Narrative Play," 24.

36 Izetta Smith, "Preschool Children 'Play' Out Their Grief," in *Death Studies* 15 (1991): 169.

37 Kopelman, "Charlotte the Spider," in *Children and Health Care: Moral and Social Issues*, eds. Loretta M. Kopelman and John C. Moskop (Boston: Kluwer Academic Publishers, 1989), 123–126.

38 Myra Bluebond-Langner, *The Private Worlds of Dying Children* (Princeton: Princeton University Press, 1980), 185.

39 V. Kudryavtsev, "The Imagination of the Preschool Child: The Experience of Logical-Psychological Analysis," in *Journal of Russian & East European Psychology* 54 (2917): 395–396.

40 Kudrayevsky, 398; For a medieval example, see Richard of St. Victor in *The Twelve Patriarchs*.

41 M. N. Bhroin, "'A Slice of Life': The Interrelationships among Art, Play and the 'Real' Life of the Young Child," in *International Journal of Education & the Arts* 8 (2997): 2.

42 Taylor, *The Language Animal*, 55.

43 G. Margherita, et al., "Invented Fairy Tales in Groups with Onco-haematological Children," in *Child: Care, Health and Development* 40 (2913): 426–427.

44 Margherita, "Invented Fairy Tales," 431.

45 Jane Peterson and Yvonne Sterling, "Children's Perceptions of Asthma: African American Children Use Metaphors to Make Sense of Asthma," in *Journal of Paediatric Health Care* (2009): 93–100.

46 Gendlin, *Experiencing*, 70.

47 Lonergan, *Insight*, 209.

48 Lonergan, *Insight*, 286.

49 Lonergan, *Insight*, 197.

50 Robert M. Doran, *Theology and the Dialectics of History* (Toronto: University of Toronto Press, 1989), 576.

51 Gendlin, *Experiencing*, 118–119.

52 Dietrich Niethammer, *Speaking Honestly with Sick And Dying Children & Adolescents: Unlocking the Silence*, trans. Victoria W. Hill (Baltimore: Johns Hopkins University Press, 2012), 114.

53 Bluebond-Langner, *Private Worlds*, 17, 165.

54 Katharina M. Ruhe, et al., "Rational Capacity: Broadening the Notion of Decision-Making Capacity in Paediatric Healthcare," *Bioethical Inquiry* 13 (2016): 518.

55 Jo-Eileen Guylay, *The Dying Child* (Toronto: McGraw-Hill, 1978), 33.

56 SickKids Toronto VS: Undeniable. https://www.youtube.com/watch?v=78mNZeDaMtk

57 From a glossary prepared by Katie MacDougald for a panel presentation at the 2021 Conference on Medicine and Religion.

58 I owe Katie MacDougald and Tyler Tate for their help in drafting this sentence.

59 Gendlin, *Experiencing*, 144–147.

60 P. van der Riet, et al., "Student Nurses Experience of a 'Fairy Garden' Healing Haven Garden for Sick Children," in *Nurse Education Today* 59 (2917): 92.

61 Smith, "Preschool Children," 174.

62 "Cities Alive: Designing for Urban Childhoods," *ARUP* December 2017.

63 Lonergan, *Insight*, 213.

CHAPTER 5

Can a Child Choose?

In Tolkien's *The Two Towers*, one of the characters, Aragorn, meets another on the grassy plains of a land called Rohan. The other character, Éomer, asks him, "What doom do you bring out of the North?" "The doom of choice," says Aragorn. "None may live now as they have lived."[1] This line comes back to me again and again as I think about parents, children, and health-care practitioners who face the myriad of complex decisions involved in caring for children with life-limiting illness. It is all well and good to talk about children as made in the image of God, about children's moral formation, about the ways in which they share our moral structures, communicate meaningfully, and make meaning in death. But this does not change the fact that in many instances, no matter how much we wish it were otherwise, concrete choices must be made.

In this chapter, I consider the question *Can a child choose?* Specifically, I am interested in what it means for a child to make a meaningful decision in the context of medical decision-making in light of their moral subjectivity and agency, and in light of the goals of childhood. I will consider where and how children are (or are not) included in medical decision-making. I will look at processes and models of making decisions together, but also at the system of medical ethics that governs the so-called difficult ethical cases. And I will approach this subject with the understanding that it reveals something about what it means for adults to make decisions, too. Children, who do not fit comfortably into the simplified models of decision-making and rationality, invite a recognition that these same models often are an obstacle to understanding adulthood.

In a 2006 article, Imelda Coyne presented her findings from a study of medical consultations with children in hospital: Children's own views were underused, and their participation relied on how cognitively mature health-care professionals (in this case nurses) judged them to be.[2] Specifically, children's involvement in their own care often depended on whether they were seen as being rational subjects, a judgment tightly tied to their age. Some readers complained that the findings were unoriginal and pointless because we all know children are insufficiently consulted. But, as both Coyne and a paper respondent, Jolley, pointed out, for most of our society, the opposite is true. While it may be common knowledge among pediatric researchers that children are insufficiently involved in their own care, the general assumption within and without medicine is that children *are* being consulted, because their right to participation is enshrined in government policies and hospital initiatives. Coyne's research demonstrated that what is enshrined in policy does not bear out in practice.

We should then ask *why?* In many ways, this question has driven this entire book. Why aren't children who are dying informed, consulted, involved in decision-making, and referred to palliative care? What assumptions do we make about who children are, the nature and goals of childhood, and about death, and what role do these assumptions play in children's participation in their medical care and in their dying? Why isn't a peaceful death as much a goal as a cure or the prevention of premature death? On what grounds and with what assumptions about moral reasoning do we determine a child's capacity to participate in these decisions? These are vital questions for exactly the reasons Coyne's study demonstrated: Even though there is tacit agreement that children should be included in medical decision-making, there is little evidence that this is becoming widespread practice, let alone in a way that deeply thinks about what it means for children to be moral subjects and agents who make meaning in their lives, who communicate their experiences, and who transform themselves, those around them, and the world.

***

One reason for this failure to ask the deeper questions, I think, is that policy is inherently practical and based on preconceived notions of common sense, so it rarely questions underlying ideas about children, language, death, and hospital structures, which reinforce the marginalization of children. I suggest that a significant reason why children are so often excluded from decision-making, and why—despite the general recognition that they have a right to participation—their views are underused and undervalued, is because our models of decision-making in medicine, like those of moral agency more generally, are *predicated on adult goals, defined by adult structures, and hold adults as the model of rationality.* As with most moral frameworks for decision-making, the framework of decision-making in pediatric settings has simply adapted adult models and outcomes to the pediatric setting, making adjustments to account for the extra stakeholders.

When I say that children's participation is predicated on adult goals, I mean this in several ways. First, one repeated goal of involving children in decision-making is expressed as helping them develop into rational, autonomous decision-makers.[3] That is, children should be included in light of what they will one day become. Second, the goals of individual decisions are generally also set by adults. That is, the decision is presented by adults, the options outlined by adults, and the correct or rational choice is often predetermined by adults. The threshold for determining rationality is often made based on "the stance that the choice of a mature child would be the same as that of an adult."[4] In other words, the child is viewed as capable when she makes the decision an adult would make. The prevalence of this assumption is borne out in the evidence that health-care professionals are less likely to take a child's view seriously when the child disagrees with the proposed plan of action.[5] Third, adults generally decide on the appropriate amount of information a child can receive. This should be an obvious statement, but children's participation in decision-making requires communication. If parents are unwilling to talk with their children about the child's impending death, their silence will necessarily limit the ability for children to participate in end-of-life decision-making.

Children's participation is also defined by adult structures. Decision-making models in pediatric care are often simply adapted from models for adult patient care. For example, in an article on Shared Decision-Making (SDM), currently the standard for good medical decision-making, researchers adapt a diagram from adult SDM to the pediatric setting. In place of the adult patient, this new diagram depicts a parent-child dyad.[6] The child does not exist as a dialogue partner in her own right but is simply bundled with the parent. Neither the role of the parents nor the role of the child, nor their relationship to each other, is clearly defined. Children's participation is also affected by the environmental and interpersonal structures in which decision-making takes place. Lin, et al., found that hospital systems had a significant impact on decision-making; parents often felt forced into certain decisions, or had to make a decision on an inappropriate time-scale, due to the scheduling needs of health-care providers.[7] This conclusion is consistent with studies of children's participation more generally, which find that the structures of the hospital system inhibit children's ability to be adequately informed and to have the chance to participate.[8] In contrast to a hospital's regimented and scheduled consultations, research suggests that children prefer to participate in more informal modes of communication.[9] Parents of children should not be surprised by this: How many times have you sat your child down to have a serious talk about something only to find that she resolutely resists hearing about it and giving her opinion? However, at some other moment, she will often unexpectedly blurt out her views on the topic. Naturally, this will be at the most inconvenient time for her parents. In other words, children want to be able to make decisions in their own way at their own pace.

Yet in hospital settings, children are expected to solve problems in an adult manner.[10] A recurring theme in all discussions of children's participation in medical decision-making is whether they are sufficiently rational. Children's participation is significantly impacted by the judgment of health-care professionals regarding the child's rationality, and so implicit or explicit beliefs about children's rationality held by these professionals are, in practice, one of the most important barriers to children's participation in decision-making.[11] As I will discuss later in this chapter, this extends to concerns about children's abilities for meaningful participation, where meaningful is defined according to particular rational capacities. In this case, "rationality is no more than inferential reasoning, and morality is no more than a rational moral theory."[12] The rational adult manner envisions decision-making as a straightforward process, where problems are identified, rationally deliberated, and a solution chosen and verbally justified in a reasonable manner. Children's ability to make decisions is measured against this.

The research into SDM in the pediatric setting is particularly telling.[13] In general, findings suggest that shared decision-making in cases involving children have trouble moving past the decision-maker–physician dyad to properly include all of the relevant decision-makers, including the patient, their family, and their health-care practitioners. In addition, the findings suggest that most decisions are not shared, but are either autonomous or paternalistic, meaning that ultimately, either the parent or the physician decides what to do. In addition, many "shared" decisions really involve the physician communicating with the families to have them align their decision with what the physician believes to be the best, rather than being a truly shared endeavor where all of the participants shape the process and results. Studies of SDM in cases involving children confirm that while "everyone" agrees that children should participate in decision-making, very few of them do in reality, even accounting for cases where their illness is severe enough to prevent participation. Finally, the SDM models used in the studies generally simplify the process of decision-making and underestimate the number of people involved in the process.

Most concerningly, however, research into children's participation—even by researchers who are dedicated to including children in their own medical care—often fails to break out of these adult-driven categories. In an otherwise excellent article on children's participation in medical decision-making, Jeremic states that children who are too young to attend school are unable to participate because they do not possess "sufficient cognitive capacities to understand and comprehend medical information."[14] But why not? He leaves unquestioned what accounts of capacity he assumes. His conclusion is simply not borne out in other studies on children's comprehension, for example on children's abilities to play out traumatic events, or Nova's study discussed in the previous chapter on children's communication in a clinical setting.[15] Elsewhere, a study of shared decision-making finds that research into interventions to improve participation in pediatric SDM "rarely targeted patients (i.e., children) but focused mainly on parents . . . with only 7 percent of interventions targeting the pediatric patient alone and 19 percent targeting the pediatric patient with another party."[16] To prevent children from participating in medical decision-making based on preconceived ideas about their abilities will become a self-fulfilling prophecy.

Children's participation in institutional settings, then, is often initiated and governed by adults, and tends to "mirror or imitate adult models of participation."[17] Children depend upon adults for the legitimacy of their actions in that sphere and rarely have any say in the larger institutional aims and structures. Yet models for shared decision-making that do not question the principlist moral systems, individualist measurements of capacity, and primacy of literal speech in medicine, will never be able to properly engage children. We must ask, then, whether children are unable to participate because they inherently lack the capacity to do so, or because the structures around them prevent their participation. Similar questions are addressed in social models of disability, which locate disability not in the individual but in structures that are inherently disabling. For example, what is disabling is not legs that do not move on their own, but the lack of access to wheelchairs, or the lack of wheelchair access to buildings, public transit, and homes.[18]

Hospitals, like schools, churches, subways, and courtrooms, are not immune from their cultural surroundings. As the first two chapters of this book suggested, prevailing cultural ideas about children and their abilities have a significant influence on these institutions. Not only that, but these institutions themselves create their own cultures, which in turn incubate their own accepted decision-making models and moral theories. These institutions also operate according to preconceived notions about who and what is a human being. In Coyne's study, children put into their own words a recurring critique of the biomedical model: that they were made to feel like pieces of meat, like objects to be manipulated, rather than whole persons.[19] In order to open up spaces for children—who are not pieces of meat, but moral agents who can meaningfully express their experiences and make meaning even in the face of death—to participate in medical decision-making, we must transform institutional structures that have traditionally excluded them.

This transformation of structures means rethinking the goals and models of rationality in medical decision-making from a childist perspective, such as the one I have laid out in this book. The preceding chapters demonstrate that children are capable of meaningfully expressing what it is that they want. The fact that children and adults share in the same moral world as each other means that this agency can be shared. Against a principlist view modeled on a binary relationship between patient and physician, then, I advocate for an approach that sees decision-making as a shared venture which is part of the broader moral formation and agency of children. In this larger view, meaning is communicative. This communication can proceed asymmetrically; a child can communicate at the level of experience or desire, and an adult can interpret this in terms of a judgment and return the formulation to the child for confirmation. In this way, we can have meaningful shared decision-making. In exploring the moral agency that is grounded in the prior "we" of intersubjectivity, and involves communicative acts of meaning, we can move away from highly individualized accounts of decision-making in favor of a meaningful shared model. In this account of shared decision-making, we do not only take into account different views or opinions, but also value different strengths, abilities, and ways of being in the world.

As I mentioned in the introduction, pediatric medicine is one of the few places focused on the questions of children's meaningful participation in decision-making, and one of the institutions in which the commitment to children's participation is most obvious. As a moral theologian interested in children's agency, it is interesting to me that so much of the material I find about children's actual participation in moral decision-making, and about their moral agency in general, comes out of medical literature. Medical situations force us to confront the issue of children's participation in a way that is simply more pressing than in so many other aspects of life.

However, this also means that much of what we learn in pediatrics about involving children in decision-making never makes it out of the hospitals and into society in general. This is a missed opportunity, because the complexities of pediatric decision-making are also valuable in what they reveal about the inclusion of children *outside* the hospital, and how we truly do make decisions at any age.[20] The reality is that decision-making in the medical setting rarely serves the needs of adults either, or adequately allows parents and/or adult patients to make truly informed and shared decisions. Most adults involve others in their decision-making, and act as persons in relationship, rather than as a rational individual free from external influence and constraint.

Thus, in this chapter, I argue that children can meaningfully participate in decision-making, because they are moral subjects and agents—even children who are significantly limited in cognitive and communicative abilities. This type of participation is interpersonal and grounded in shared meaning rather than in abstract principles or individualized rationality. It requires us to reconsider a child's capacity for comprehension and decision-making and reexamine who in the life of a child has a right to be involved in decision-making processes. Here, I am especially interested in the place we give to siblings. If child-centered care is also family-centered care, and children should be allowed to participate, then I suggest that siblings should be included as decision-makers. Finally, I argue that this model invites a reconsideration of our structures for adult decision-making, based on the childist account of human morality I have laid out in this book.

Children are capable of meaningful participation in decision-making. We are thus obliged to creatively think about how to support and nurture their collaboration, whether by increasing direct communication with children, limiting adult speech, researching and implementing various nonverbal tools, and improving health-care providers' and parents' ability to communicate with children at appropriate levels. Including children in medical decision-making is challenging in many ways, not least in the sheer time and effort it takes to find effective ways of communicating with them. We can think of the need for this effort as akin to requiring a translator when treating a patient who speaks a foreign language—except, in this case, we ourselves must learn this new tongue. In the second chapter, I highlighted the ways in which moral agency is akin to a skill that must be learned. Children need to be taught and their developing ethical intentionality nurtured, but we must undertake this endeavor on a level in which they can understand and engage.

However, and I want to make this very clear, I am not suggesting that children, because they are moral subjects and agents, should be making these decisions *alone*. Nor am I suggesting that the goal of involving children in decision-making is to help them become autonomous moral agents, although moral development is an important aspect of children's participation. Seeing decision-making as a shared venture requires adults to critically reflect on their decisions, and integrate insights and questions put forward by the child or children involved; in these ways it helps to mitigate issues of bias but also acknowledges the need of children to decide in community. Importantly, since moral agency is formed in part by experience, the chance to be included in medical decision-making should not be sprung on children at the end of life but be integrated from their first encounters with the medical system.

This chapter cannot completely reimagine the medical system and its decision-making and ethical models. But I do want to sketch out some of its barriers to children's participation and make modest remedial proposals based on the work of this book. This chapter is an invitation for those directly involved in pediatric care to think beyond the hospital system, about what children reveal about our moral personhood and structures in a way that does not simply adapt adult structures for children. It is also an invitation for those who are not pediatric specialists to consider what it means for children to make decisions, and to make decisions that are properly shared. The medical system exists within webs of culture, and children's participation requires not only a medical system in which they can participate. They need to be trained, encouraged, and prepared in life in general. Inasmuch as decision-making is a skill, they need training and development. In essence, for children to participate fully in pediatric decision-making, they need to be recognized as moral agents in all elements of their lives.

Pediatric decision-making, especially when facing death, is incredibly complex, for multiple reasons. One is the emotional and tragic nature of so many of these decisions, which can never be fully erased through effective decision-making models and institutional support. Another is the number of people involved, each with their own views, opinions, and values. Complicating this further is the influence of all those not traditionally considered stakeholders, but with whom the stakeholders come into contact and from whom they may seek guidance, such as mentors, friends, teachers, colleagues, priests, and elders. So, when I talk about reconsidering these decision-making structures, I in no way want to pretend that this is an easy thing to do. Nor do I want to pretend that the very real medical, emotional, and cognitive limitations of children are not relevant to their participation. But just because this process is complex does not mean it should be simplified into adult-driven paradigms.

In truly shared decision-making, all stakeholders involved require support. It is hard on parents to make difficult decisions about a child's end-of-life care. It is hard on medical staff. It is hard on children. This support is also key outside of the hospital system. Properly supporting children at the end of life requires a culture that is willing to face their suffering, hear their voices, and care for them as a community. It requires us, when facing questions of end-of-life decision-making, to begin with the presumption of participation of children of all ages, from the recognition of our interpersonal and communicative moral selfhood and seek in this way to nurture their participation.

***

It is not only the practical frameworks of decision-making in medicine that present a challenge to the inclusion of children, but also the broader moral system of bioethics, which sets the foundation for these models. Tied to the lack of research into decision-making processes, the lack of interventions aimed toward children, and the persistent notion that children below school age are incapable of participation, is the principlist moral system at work in the hospital system, which views autonomy as the foundation and goal of human moral participation. This system is what Margaret Urban Walker describes as a theoretical-juridical model of morality, which is "compact, propositionally codifiable, impersonally action-guiding, [and based on a] set of law-like propositions."[21] In other words, it is a "purified code of moral knowledge."

It is within this system, with its particular account of impersonal rationality, that we find sentiments that children's imagination and emotionality (that is, how they are so often governed by their feelings) inhibit their ability to rationally participate in medical decision-making. This concern extends to parents as well: "A barrier to rational decision making for parents, as well as other stakeholders, is the emotionally charged nature of many medical decisions."[22] Tied to this account of impersonal rationality is also an implicit skepticism that children can meaningfully participate in decision-making. But as I have talked about, feelings are apprehensions of value. They are *part of* our ethical intentionality, not a barrier. And as I discussed in chapter 4, children are meaningful communicators. How, then, do we square children's true capacities with the structures of which they are a part?

Contemporary bioethics in North America takes a principlist approach, and this is true also in pediatric bioethics.[23] In this section, then, I will examine the principlist approach and its concerns about the meaningfulness of children's participation, focusing on the way this assumption informs moral systems that exclude children. As I will show, these systems only seem reasonable because they do not attempt to include children and refuse to allow their ethical intentionality to transform our understanding of morality and decision-making.

Childress and Beauchamp's four principles of bioethics, first articulated in their 1979 book *Principles of Bioethics*, now form the bedrock of medical ethics: autonomy, beneficence, nonmaleficence, and justice. The reasons for these particular principles, as well perhaps as the principlist approach in general, are historical; the origins of bioethics are not in patient care or physician-patient relationships *per se*, but rather in medical research. Bioethics as its own field originated in North America in response to several instances of medical research undertaken without consent, most famously the Tuskegee Syphilis Study. In response to these events, the United States government got significantly involved in the medical field for the first time, issuing the Belmont Report, which among other things introduced three guiding moral principles for medical research: autonomy (i.e., informed consent), beneficence, and justice. The approach taken in the report is characterized by a prioritization of individual rights and moral minimalism; there is little consideration of the goods of medicine or the relationship between medicine and the moral life.[24]

Pediatric bioethics does not differ significantly from this approach, except that it is common for pediatric bioethics to rearrange or increase the number of principles in light of the complexities involved in making medical decisions for children, not least because of the acknowledgment that children lack the autonomy to decide for themselves. This reliance on principles dictates how ethical situations are presented, debated, and settled in pediatric bioethics. In this principlist framework, ethical situations are solved by the application of principles, ethical problems arise when one or more principles is in conflict, and ethical resolution comes from adjudicating which principle is most pertinent to the given situation.[25] We can find an example of this approach in Carter's *Palliative Care for Infants, Children, and Adolescents*, in which the chapter on conflict resolution "aims to improve the way ethical questions related to palliative care are addressed in order to optimize the effectiveness of care provided to the child and family."[26] To do this, the chapter lays out six principles, called "core values" by the authors, which are foundational to the patient–health-care provider relationship: beneficence, nonmaleficence, autonomy, fidelity, respect for life, and respect for persons.

This principlist approach is lacking in several ways. First, while in pediatric approaches to bioethics beneficence comes to take precedence over autonomy, the framework is still predicated on autonomy. The reason beneficence takes precedence in pediatrics is the conviction that children are incapable of making medical decisions. With little substantive criteria for beneficence, however, it is unclear how this principle functions, except that the autonomous subject changes from the patient to the surrogate decision-maker. In all other areas of bioethics, autonomy dominates; in North America especially, autonomy has eclipsed all other principles as the guiding principle for ethical medical care. The dominance of autonomy is tied to the procedural account of moral decision-making; it is the fact that the decision is "mine" that makes it moral.

In the case of children, they cannot make decisions that are properly "theirs" because they lack capacity. But beneficence presents a different issue. Beneficence, functionally defined as that which is in the best interest of the patient, presumably has substantive commitments: that is, there must be some criteria for what is or is not in the best interests of a child in order to effectively implement this principle. But who decides what these criteria are? In fraught cases, it often comes down to the autonomy of the parents or the autonomy of the physicians to decide what is in the best interest of the child. Further, it is unclear how we apply a particular principle or arbitrate between two or three principles in conflict. If there are no rules governing which principle is applied to which situation, or how we describe the inherent conflict in a given situation, we are left with the unpalatable conclusion that much of morality is arbitrary or substantiated only by autonomous fiat.

Third, this seemingly simple approach to ethics masks a considerable problem—that it is complex in practice. How do we even know what a principle means? It can be a matter of principle that we do not lie, but to follow this principle one must know what a lie is.[27] But there is an even deeper problem, as Hoffmaster illustrates: "how do we decide whether a 'given principle' is relevant to a 'given course of action,' and indeed, how do we determine what the relevant description of a 'given course of action' is?"[28] Answering those questions is no easy task, and a principlist framework does not give us the resources to answer them. Descriptions of situations and the decisions to be made are also shaped by the values of those who present the issue. In the basic model for shared decision-making, Chris Feudtner et al., argue that decision-making is commonly presented as several solutions to one problem, where this problem is defined by clinicians.[29] Unclear too are the goals shaping such presentations of solutions. If we think of cure or the prolongation of life as the goal of treatment decisions, for example, the way we present these goals will be fundamentally different than if we deem a peaceful death an equally valued goal.

But even more alarming to me is the deeply impersonal character of this principlist approach, which stands in contrast to the childist account of ethical intentionality developed in the second chapter. Of special concern is the way that it erases the subject of the moral conflict. One of the biggest deficiencies in the common approach to bioethics is that the patient, in this case a child, is forgotten in the midst of these ethical conundrums, because situations are characterized as conflicts between two or more health-care principles. Arguably, it also forgets parents and health-care professionals, because they are not seen as self-transcendent subjects but merely as arbitrators between two principles. In this model, the key to solving a dilemma is to figure out which principle takes precedent in the given situation, to the exclusion of the moral person.

For example, Carter's palliative care handbook presents two ethical dilemmas involving children who are old enough to speak and are capable of interaction—one a seven-year-old with leukemia, and another a ten-year-old with a brain tumor—but mentions neither the children's opinions, values, thoughts, desires, or wishes, nor their experience of illness, hospitalization, or treatment. The chapter does not specify that these conflicts involve a relationship between the child, the parents, and the health-care team; most of the scenarios presented in the chapter consider the health-care professionals and parents only.

In essence, then, the standard model of the physician-patient relationship has simply been shifted to the physician–parent relationship, with no consideration that involving a child may require a new and different framework. Due to its focus on the adults and the principles, the child in question is forgotten. This oversight is reflected in the lacuna of research I mentioned earlier in this chapter on children's ability to make decisions in a medical setting, nor is there much evidence for attempts at truly shared decision-making. Children, when asked, express a desire to be included and consulted in decisions involving their medical care, but "in practice, children are often not given a real opportunity to participate in decisions."[30] A 2007 study interviewing children between the ages of six and eleven found that "30 percent indicated they were not adequately informed" about their medical procedures and "61 percent did not have a chance to participate in decision-making."[31] Another study published in the same year which considered children's acute care visits concluded that 65 percent of children had a passive role in their medical care consultations.[32]

One of the key worries that permeates medical literature on children's participation in decision-making is about children's ability to *meaningfully* participate. This is a concern in both the principlist bioethics and medical decision-making more generally. Both systems are built on the same foundation, which assumes the application of abstract knowledge (of medical or moral principles, in this case) to a given situation. What makes a decision meaningful is rarely explicitly defined, but can be roughly characterized as two, sometimes connected, criteria. One is that a meaningful choice arises from the ability to select values and preferences, and act according to them. Many articles talk about young or severely compromised children as having no known values, wishes, preferences, feelings—what McCabe, et al., describe as "purely subjective factors and values."[33] Meaningful decisions, then, can signify decisions that are in accordance with the subject's values and preferences. But other times, the term is used to mean a "reasonable choice," a choice that most rational people would also make.[34] For Childress and Beauchamp, the ability to make meaningful decisions is grounded in a rational capacity for judgment, to act "freely in accordance with a self-chosen plan."[35] Similarly, Luc Bovens describes rational capacity as the capacity for discernment.[36] As I mentioned earlier, Jeremic, et al., claim that "most children of pre-school age (younger than five to six years) do not possess a sufficient level of comprehension to meaningfully participate in decision-making."[37] Ernst, et al., make reference to patients who are not able to participate meaningfully in decision-making but offer no definition or corresponding capabilities required for meaningful participation.[38] Ruhe, et al., note that in bioethics, "decision-making capacity denotes a person's ability to make choices."[39]

What these approaches do not make clear, though, is what makes something meaningful instead of meaningless. Children are said to lack the rational capabilities needed to make meaningful decisions and are thus denied participation in decisions involving their medical care. But the definition of meaningful here is unclear—meaningful as opposed to arbitrary? To insubstantial? To meaningless? The failure in bioethics literature to clearly articulate what is a meaningful decision means that thought around these issues focuses entirely on the procedural capacity for making choices and not on meaning. This is true also in shared decision-making initiatives. Further, responses to this lacuna that argue for children's participation in medical decision-making suffer from the same lack of clarity regarding what is intended by "meaningful," and have trouble explaining that while children should participate in decision-making, it is inappropriate for them to be making the entirety of their health-care decisions alone.[40]

The exclusion of children on the basis of their perceived lack of ability to make meaningful decisions is based on a confusion over what meaning is, and how it relates to judgment. As I argued in chapter 4, the view that children are too immature, or simply unable, to express their viewpoints is tied to particular beliefs about language and the capacities necessary for truthful expression. I argued against the enframing theory of language, and instead posited that the meaningfulness of children's experience is generated in their attempts to symbolize it, both to themselves and to others, and is brought to fruition in back-and-forth communication with others in which the experience is further symbolized and interpreted. That is, this communication is interpersonal and shared. Speech, as well as gesture and other nonverbal symbols, is wrapped up in a shared endeavor to understand, and is not simply a contextless expression of children's interior thoughts and experience. It relies

on the reception and creative reengagement of language and other symbolizations that are intimately tied to experience. In this view, there is no abstract
rational threshold needed for meaningful communication.

The meaningfulness of a child's experience as expressed through symbolization is not separate from judgment. Rather, meaning is tied to judgment.
When the girl in Bluebond-Langner's study made dolls and buried them in
a Kleenex box, she was not acting unreflectively, nor simply expressing her
feelings. Instead, she was revealing a judgment of fact, in this case, the fact
that she would die. This type of judgment can be brought into effective acts
of meaning; that is, judgments of value, decisions, and actions can be communicated.[41] It is these acts of meaning, it would seem, that are of concern in
bioethical literature about decision-making. Judging is another way of describing the act of making a decision on the basis of particular information that has
been weighed and tried. A judgment is reached when the relevant questions
have been asked and answered, through imagining, observing, experiencing,
testing, formulating, or any other relevant operation of rationality. Thus, it is
not a separate question of whether children can meaningfully communicate
and whether they can make meaningful decisions.

As I have argued earlier, children share in the same structure of ethical
intentionality in which we operate, where experience, reason, understanding,
and judgment are intimately related. Children are attentive to the data around
them, they reflect on their experience, they notice patterns, they make decisions and judgments, and they ask (do they ever ask) further questions. In the
collaborative approach I discussed in the previous chapter, though, children's
inchoate expressions of experience can yield judgments in a *shared* sense, where
more can be achieved collaboratively than alone. They communicate meaning,
at first intersubjectively and incarnately, but quickly maturing to be able to communicate linguistically and symbolically as well. In Bluebond-Langner's study,
drawings and making coffins for dolls were two ways children communicated
knowledge of their impending death.[42] To say then that children do not make
meaningful decisions is simply not true; because they arrive at their decisions
through observation, experience, deliberating, taking action, and so on, their
decisions are meaningful. Against the narrowness of formal reason on which
principlism is founded, understanding children as agents and originators of
meaning takes into account the creative possibilities of the moral life.[43]

Shared meaning between children and adults does not mean that they
necessarily engage in the same acts of meaning, or at the same level of

expression. Expression may have its source in experience, in a more ordered arrangement of experiences, in a statement of fact, in an act of will. In turn, the hearer or reader may respond "on the experiential level, or (2) both on the level of experience and on the level of insight and consideration, or (3) on the three levels of experience, insight, and judgment, or (4) not only on the three cognitional levels but also in the practical manner that includes an act of will."[44] A potential act of meaning made by a child may still be communicated to a parent, who can help with or complete the task of thinking, formulating, and judging. Similarly, a parent or health-care professional can help a child come to a judgment regarding the truth of what they understand about their experience. Because acts of meaning can be communicated, there is always the possibility of achieving common meaning and common judgments, not only on a societal level, but on a familial or small-group level as well.

***

As I discussed in the second section, children express a desire to participate in decisions involving their medical care but are rarely given an opportunity to do so. To address this, we must get past the binary view of decision-making as made or not made by one person, or the simplified model of contractual decision between two independent individuals and see it as a shared venture in which children have something to teach us, and we have a role in guiding them. In this way, any individual decision becomes part of a large and complex ethical intentionality, where children (and adults!) receive moral language, concepts, examples, and creatively play with them as they make their own meaning and arrive together at judgment.

Children complicate the decision-making process specifically because they are human beings who share in our moral worlds and in the goals of human life. Ethical dilemmas and medical decisions arise not because of principles or biological realities but because of persons. It is a flesh-and-blood child, not in the abstract, not as a source of conflicting principles, but in her unique humanity, who is the subject of our decisions. When we understand that meaning is deeply personal and cannot arise apart from subjects, we must change our idea of a meaningful decision—meaning is tied to particular persons and their experiences, relationships, and subjectivity. This account of meaning and judgment, and of both the abilities of children and the role of adults (including parents) in moral formation, paves the way for seeing medical decision-making as a shared venture. In moral agency that is grounded in the prior "we," and involves communicative acts of meaning, we move away from highly individualized accounts of meaning and meaningful decision-making.[45]

Contrary to an account of individual decision-making based on a narrow understanding of rationality and meaningful expression, I have argued that children can arrive at judgments of fact and value, and that these judgments can be communicated, in an inherently collaborative and asymmetrical process. Throughout this book, I have suggested that models of decision-making in medicine, like those of moral agency in general, are predicated on adult goals, defined by adult structures, and hold adults as the model of rationality. What would it look like, then, if we thought about decision-making from the perspective of child goals, child structures, and children's cognitive and ethical intentionality as included in our model of rationality? What would this mean specifically for decision-making in the medical context?

When we take a childist perspective, we see that decisions are properly shared, because children receive the moral world from others and then creatively engage with it in the asymmetrical relationships I described in chapter 2. This asymmetry means that it is the responsibility of adults to train children in the skills of decision-making, as well as to provide them with adequate support. Values, preferences, and the acquisition of knowledge are not things anyone can achieve independently. Instead, we rely on communal knowledge; adults have a conception of what is good for children and play a significant role in teaching children. On the other hand, children must learn critical reflection and they have little ability, especially at a young age, to distinguish between external commands and internal drives. The formation of their moral feelings, of their will, and of their agency requires that they are guided by others in the development of their capacities. A procedural account of capacity ignores the reality that adults, especially parents, appropriately have expectations of what a child should do and how a child should reason, and a set of values they wish to pass on to this child, not because they are co-opting her autonomy but because moral formation extends beyond the narrow confines of autonomy.[46] This also helps clarify why parents are (in almost all cases, because there are always tragic cases where parents do not love and value their children) the appropriate decision-makers for and with their children. It is parents who first share in the intersubjective encounter with their newborn, and parents who play the primary role in the formation and development of their children.

This asymmetry also means that meaning can be communicated across levels of ethical intentionality, such that an expression that is not a full judgment can be received, formulated, and possibly returned to the child for verification. But even if it cannot be verified by the child, the process of turning experience and desires into a judgment can be done collaboratively. In fact, this is something parents do all the time. Parents are so good at soothing their infant, not only because they have a familiar touch or smell, but because their methods for soothing the infant have been formed collaboratively by both the parents and child. From birth, every child has their own preferences. I recall when my daughter was five days old and crying in the night after a feed. My husband was holding her and soothing her, but to no avail. Finally, I suggested he just put her down to take a break. Instantly she stopped crying. Already she was expressing a preference to be put down awake after a night feed, a preference that has been consistent as she has aged. This is not something we trained her to do, but rather our method for caring for her arose from the relationship between her desires and our responses. Of course, our responses also shaped her desires. This was a shared, asymmetrical process.

This is just as true in the hospital setting. In a study on decision-making for children with medical complexities, researchers found that "in spite of the prevalence of neurodevelopmental delay in their children, parents consistently identified behavioral cues to the patients' preferences."[47] That is, parents paid attention to their children's expressions of meaning, symbolized here largely in bodily movements. This meaning could be considered as part of the process of arriving at judgment. In this way, the children would participate in the decision-making process even while they would not be the ones who finally arrived at a decision. But this type of communication of meaning and its relation to shared judgment needs to be properly supported in a decision-making environment. The study, interestingly, found "almost no descriptions of providers asking families about patient preferences."[48] In the shared decision-making process between parents and physicians, the physicians did not consider the children's expressions of meaning as relevant to the discussion. If these expressions are not considered, then grieving and exhausted parents must work against institutional structures in order to include their children. Many will not be able to do this.

Seeing decision-making as a shared venture requires adults to critically reflect on their decisions, to integrate insights and questions put forward by the child or children into these decisions, and to do so in a specifically childlike way. As I have argued elsewhere in this book, children's modes of knowing and expressing their knowledge do not always take the same form as adults'. They often weave in imaginative and fantastical material, and express themselves through their bodily movements, play, and art, as well as literal and nonliteral verbal expressions. Yet it is not only children who do this. Feudtner et al., critique the simplification of decision-making in all SDM models: "ethicists and decision-making experts should not consider a complex of affiliated or linked problems as extraneous or irrelevant factors intruding inappropriately upon decision making, but instead view them as part of the fabric of decision making."[49] The fact that children do not linearly proceed down one decision-making path is a reminder that *none of us do*! Feelings, "irrelevant" factors, nonmedical considerations, and so on, are properly part of how we make decisions, no matter how old we are.

In the same vein, children's reliance on others in the decision-making process is also a healthy reminder that accounts of meaningful decision-making that prioritize freedom from restraint and the interference of others, that see a binary between controlling or being controlled, ignore the ways in which we often make decisions. Decisions are rarely made immediately and are rarely made independently. Instead, decisions usually require a long dialogue with ourselves and with others. Many physicians report that they often consult their colleagues, especially when it comes to complicated cases. This is rarely noted in decision-making models. Similarly, parents and other stakeholders make their decisions in a web of relationships that include other family members, friends, religious leaders, and so on. When a choice is made, that moment is not the decision-making itself, but rather the culmination of months and perhaps years of smaller decisions, judgments, and experiences.

The shared venture approach to making decisions implies a different relationship between health-care professionals and families than the one gaining ascendency in North America. Against the view that health-care professionals are service providers to whom we make demands, children, parents, and health-care providers must see growing in understanding and coming to judgment as a joint venture. This requires humility on all sides: There is already a shift in the medical community to inform and include children, but physicians often face pushback from parents.[50] Parental concerns should not be seen as impediments to care, but as opportunities to forge closer relationships. This approach is gaining traction in pediatrics, as numerous studies testify to the closeness between families and care providers, and the many ways in which families rely on health-care professionals for comfort and guidance. Furthermore, children have a significant amount to teach doctors about what it means to practice medicine, through the ways in which children are capable of shaping the therapeutic alliance, and how interactions with children shape the lives of physicians by making moral demands on them.

Approaching decision-making as a shared venture also changes what it means to assess capacity. The theory of language I discussed in the previous chapter, and the moral theory I discussed in chapter 2, suggest that a capacity evaluation for children must be done differently, and that our understanding of "shared" in shared decision-making must be different. We should then think of capacity not in general, nor even for this or that particular decision, which is how capacity is generally defined in hospitals. Instead, assessments of capacity should arise within the communicative context of the particular child, health-care professionals, and family, and the extent to which the child can acquire the necessary cognitive and emotional skills in collaboration with others.

To see how this can look in practice, let us look to a fictional example. In *At the Back of the North Wind*, between Diamond's two bouts of illness, his father loses his job as a gentleman's coachman, and works instead as a cabbie.[51] At one point, he falls ill and is unable to work. Facing poverty, Diamond decides to work in his father's place. He gets up the first day and goes to harness the horse, which is significantly larger than him. The harness is heavy and difficult to manage. Worried that his efforts will be met by disapproval, he works alone and creatively figures out, with the help of the obedient horse, how to get all the straps in place. The other cabbies witness this and encourage him. They also check the harness and straps when he is done to make sure that it is done correctly. As he goes out to drive, some clients recognize him and his horse, and ask after his father. Other fares (and a policeman) ask him to prove his driving abilities and his knowledge of pricing. At one point, a cabbie unconnected with him harasses him, and he is saved from trouble by a drunken cabman he has befriended previously. When he returns home in the evening, one of the other cabbies offers to unharness and feed the horse so that Diamond can eat and go to bed.

So, we can ask the question: Does Diamond have the capacity to work as a cabbie? If we ask before we let him try, our answer is likely to be no. Diamond is young and small for his age. If we focus only on Diamond's biologically unfolding qualities, as it were, such as his young age, lack of height, and lack of strength, we will not think he can do it. If we focus on what Diamond can achieve all by himself, we are no likelier to be convinced. Even though he can manage to harness the horse properly, it is a significant undertaking that he would be unlikely to be able to repeat day in and day out. If we ask in the abstract what a child like Diamond—that is, any given child—can do in the absence of support, then his capacity is definitely in doubt. But Diamond is not just any child, and his capacity needs to be considered in light of who he is in his context. The fact that Diamond is capable relies on many factors— previous experience working alongside his father, a horse that is well-trained and obedient, and other cabbies to check his work and help him in the future. In the same way, when we consider a child's ability to participate in decision-making, we need to consider what is true of that child in her context.

This example highlights another inescapable feature of end-of-life decision-making for children: While Diamond is able to work thanks to the help of others, we can still acknowledge that his situation is far from perfect. In an ideal world, Diamond would not have to work to save his family from ruin. Likewise, in an ideal world, children would not have to face death or make difficult decisions about their end-of-life care. If we focus on idealizations of childhood, children should not have to work to support their parents, so we may want to answer the question of Diamond's labor before we even consider his capacity. In this same way, some people want to shield children from a knowledge of death and it is this, not capacity, that determines whether they let children participate in end-of-life decision-making. But we have little control over these circumstances: Instead of focusing on the way in which dying is contrary to what we wish for childhood, we should instead focus on how to help children in their situation.

Viewing decision-making as a shared venture in line with the childist account of ethical intentionality also invites a reconsideration of bias. In Childress and Beauchamp's chapter on autonomy, for example, they present a binary between controlling or being controlled. The autonomous person is free from control, whereas "a person of diminished autonomy . . . is in some respect controlled by others."[52] That is, either a person is autonomous, or she is biased—controlled—by other members of the decision-making process. Children, however, have less ability to creatively engage with the moral notions, examples, and patterns that they have inherited. They have less sophisticated moral paradigms, a narrower range of examples and cases, and a less developed ethical intentionality. They need help to reach a decision.

But attending to human morality from a childist perspective, we can also see that this need is continuous in us as adults; we are always constituted by others. Even as adults we receive the moral world from others and engage with it from within a network of preexisting relationships that shape what we think. Our desires are always wrapped up with others' because we are intersubjective and interpersonal subjects. In this sense, according to the autonomy-based account, we are all "biased."

To overcome bias, then, is not to free ourselves from the influence of others. Instead, we need to constantly reflect, to ask and answer further questions about the situation and what we can do. We need the inbreaking of new meaning. In this account, bias is the prevention of asking and answering further questions in order to arrive at a reasonable judgment, in a process where feelings are integral to ethical intentionality, rather than viewed as interfering with reason. Including children in decision-making will help parents and guardians make choices that properly take into account the experiences of the child patient. Bias is harder to maintain when children are involved—they have an uncanny and often annoying habit of asking those further questions.

If bias limits moral creativity by refusing insights and stopping questions, then uncovering bias and encouraging questions is certainly an important step toward developing new ways of decision-making alongside children. While their abilities may limit the extent of their participation, children can always bring meaning to decisions, even if only by awakening new acts of meaning in their parents and caregivers. The fact that people have psychological baggage, that individuals and groups act in their own self-interest to the detriment of others, and that our values influence our experiences and judgments, makes it vital for us to question mistaken optimism, love, or heroism that obfuscates the real and necessary boundaries to ethical human action, and reminds us that to act in another's best interest means putting into question our own interests. But excluding children, and especially excluding their own version of their experiences and understanding, makes it unlikely that we will have asked and answered all relevant questions about a child's medical care. This is especially the case in the few but real instances where parents do not act in the best interests of their children, or when physicians do not act in the best interests of their patients. Childlikeness always has something to teach us, if only nothing more than the narrowness of our adult views.

Still, in the end, it is parents who have the right as surrogate decision-makers to decide for their children. Part of the issue here is that basic models of informed consent and shared decision-making "assume that each surrogate has a stable set of values and preferences that can be drawn out and applied to the decision,"[53] and that these values are separable from the surrogate's roles as a parent, a spouse, etc. But how we view the task of parenting will certainly influence our decision-making on behalf of children. Parents of children with life-limiting illness sometimes feel that they have already failed in their parental duty to protect their child. "This may lead parents to decide, based on their rubric of what would constitute being a 'good parent,' that a 'good parent' never gives up."[54] Similarly, physicians are often under pressure, internally or externally, to be able to save the child from death, or to view their death as a failure. At the end of a child's life, the inability on the part of anyone involved to acknowledge the reality that the child is dying will inevitably bias decision-making.

There is a difference between predicating the right of children to participate on their (rational) capabilities, and appropriately evaluating and responding to their particular abilities and limitations. While a child's participation in decision-making, especially the weight given to their opinions and desires, will still be determined by their abilities, our obligation to include them does not arise because of their abilities but because of their humanity. Children should be included in decision-making precisely because they are subjects and moral agents. Their inclusion should not be a way of achieving predefined goals or treatment plans, but on the basis that this is morally appropriate to who children are. Children are "willful, purposeful individuals capable of creating their own world, as well as acting in the world others create for them."[55] Children will bring new meaning to these decisions. They may not make the final decision or even all of the decisions, but they can meaningfully participate in that process.

One corollary to our obligation to extend participation rights to children is that we should also include siblings in decision-making. Siblings are frequently forgotten in pediatric care, both in formal decision-making structures and in research into their experiences and their role in caring for their ill brother or sister. Many frameworks acknowledge that siblings have a vested interest in the situation, but they have few to no rights to participation in medical decision-making. Siblings (and other nonparental family members) are rarely found in charts of decision-makers, though they may be listed as stakeholders.

But in a shared account of moral decision-making, siblings help to shape the moral world, often share special communication with their siblings in modes that differ from their parents', and, like any child, wake new meanings and invite a reconsideration of the goals of the human life. They challenge bias by asking and answering further questions. As such, they should be included.

We include children—patients and siblings alike—because of who they already are, not because of who they will become.

∗

Children can wake meanings where we do not see them, leading us to reconsider the situation and see the possibility for different judgments. Further, including children in the decision-making process serves as a constant reminder of the subject of the decision: Medical dilemmas about care for children are not some abstract battle of principles but are about the life of a person. Children, as moral subjects and agents who meaningfully participate in decision-making, ought to be included in medical decision-making, and their complex ethical intentionality should reshape decision-making goals and models within medical care. We should begin with a presumption of participation for children of all ages. But what does this mean in practice? I do not specialize in communication with children in a medical setting, but here I offer several suggestions for what these new models and goals might look like.

First, presuming children's participation means beginning any design of medical decision-making models, patient-physician interaction, or hospital spaces from the position that children's communication is meaningful and that children are moral agents who meaningfully participate. Thus, children should (like adults) have to prove their incapacity to participate, rather than having to prove their capacity. These new designs would entail training physicians and other health-care providers, as well as parents, to attend to children's expressions and symbolizations, and to view these as inherently meaningful, both in structured meetings but also in more casual encounters. We should question why and on what basis we bring preconceived ideas about which is the correct decision for a child to make. That is, we should take children's rejection of a proposed course of action as seriously as their approval.

This presumption should extend to research as well. Many of the researchers on whose work I have depended advocate for more research and less dependence on a priori models. But research about children's ability to make decisions always operates according to some model with its own latent assumptions about decision-making and rational capacity. We should ground this research in a childist account of ethical intentionality that takes children seriously as moral subjects and agents. I think this research should extend beyond pediatrics to medical decision-making more generally, to find what children reveal to us about our own embedded relationality.

The presumption of participation and the changing assessment of capacity should invite us to consider the interventions and tools we provide to children. If it is a particular child in her context that determines capacity, and her context can be changed through supportive structures, then we need to ensure we give to her and foster the supportive structures that enable her to express her ethical intentionality. Consider again the example of Diamond working as a cabbie. We can ask: If Diamond succeeded in large part because his father exposed him to methods of harnessing a horse, in what ways are we preparing children to participate in moral decision-making? We could also ask: Do our structures make children feel the need to hide their efforts, in the way Diamond harnessed the horse in secret? We must normalize the involvement of children in decision-making and moral reflection both within and without the hospital. Researchers note that one of the barriers in including children in SDM is that parents are unused to involving their children in decisions more generally.[56] Diamond would not have been able to take over driving a cab from his father without prior knowledge and skill; similarly, children will be less capable of making decisions without prior training.

However, a child's context should not be deterministic. In cases where a child has insufficient capacity due to lack of decision-making and communication skills or has been historically uninvolved, within pediatric medicine we should consider the interventions and tools aimed at children, parents, and health-care providers that can help to overcome these limitations. For example, researchers cite young children's inability to understand medical information as one reason why they cannot participate in medical decision-making. But studies of children in the medical setting have found that physicians overestimate the efficacy of their communication, and many children report that information was not given to them at an appropriate level. Thus, improving communication about medical information, possibly through mixed media—that is, not only through verbal means but using artistic or imaginative methods as well—would improve the capacity of children to participate in decision-making. Their capacity is not fixed, but determined by personal, interpersonal, and contextual factors.

Diamond's ability to harness and drive the cab also depended on having a space in which to do so: The barn provided physical structures to support him as well as a space for him to encounter other cabbies who ended up helping him. In a similar way, we should think about creating spaces where children can participate in decision-making in more collaborative and informal modes. I am thinking here of the possibilities that might exist in fairy gardens and other play spaces where children, parents, and health-care professionals can connect away from the pressures of treatment-specific places. Similarly, the fairy tale storytelling groups described in the previous chapter might be expanded to include other family members and perhaps even nurses and physicians. We should consider what possibilities exist in those sorts of spaces for both spontaneous and structured expression of desires. Fairy tales have been shown to be a way that children can talk about death and make meaning. Why could they not be a way to explore possible courses of treatment? It is quite possible that a child is more empowered to tell the story of a fairy tale character who decides to accept death than she is to express this in a decision-making conversation when the physician rounds.

In these spaces, children can be encountered as whole persons, and their participation in decision-making at the end of life can become part of a larger set of decisions to be made and meaning to be created. That is, these spaces open up the possibilities of integrating into end-of-life care the so-called nonmedical decisions, like funeral planning, saying goodbye to friends and family, choosing a preferred place of death, and so forth. That is, to care for children who are dying, and to help prepare them for death, requires that we think creatively about how to create space for all that matters to a child at the end of life.

These parallels to Diamond's story are not perfect, because there is in his context one proper way to harness a horse and one proper way to drive a cab. That is, the goals or outcomes are predetermined in his case. But when it comes to decision-making at the end of life, children should also have a say in what their goals are. Giving them the means to do so means adjusting decision-making models to recognize that a child is not just a part of a parent-child dyad but a meaningful communicator and decision-maker in her own right. Having a specific place for a child in a decision-making framework is one way to ensure that the child's views are always sought. This model presumes input from children and works hard to get it, even while recognizing that, especially in the case of children with life-limiting illness, their ability to communicate may be severely limited. Such models should also express the reality that all decisions are shared, and that all decision-making is convoluted, so the fact that children's participation is less linear is not an inherent problem.

Finally, because children's selfhood is constituted by others through shared language and moral imitation, we must accept that what a child wants is never fully separable from her context. We will never know which part of a child's desires is "truly her own" and which is another's, since all of her desires are shaped by others. In a discussion around shared decision-making in the *Toronto Star*, an ethicist at SickKids Hospital in Toronto talked about the complexities of understanding a child's wishes. "When a twelve-year-old was asked if he would have a second lung transplant for cystic fibrosis, he said, 'I would have to, or my mother would be so disappointed.' How do you tease out what he's really feeling versus his role in the family? For us to try to get to the voice of the child is very complex."[57] But this ethicist is setting up two things in opposition to each other: what the child is *really* feeling versus the duties and responsibilities that he feels toward his family. But who this child is *in his family* is inseparably part of who he is, and thus his desire not to disappoint a parent is legitimate. We can and should encourage him to talk with his parents about this decision— would they really be disappointed if he chose to forgo a second transplant, for example? If so, why? But we need to escape a framework that implies that children (or anyone) have desires that are properly their own, free from the influence of their relationships. The child's desire to care for his parents is part of his ethical intentionality.

Involving children in decision-making also has demonstrable practical benefits. McCabe notes that compliance among teenagers who participate in their medical decision-making is much higher; they feel more in control of their situation and therefore more comfortable with it.[58] It prevents children from being dependent on their own guesswork and fantasies about their condition and prognosis.[59] Furthermore, involving children in their care decisions means that parents and care providers do not have to constantly lie to children. This is an issue of considerable importance to children, for whom trust and truth-telling are especially closely related.[60] Involving children in decisions surrounding their medical care helps to combat the fear, loneliness, and isolation that has otherwise characterized children's dying in hospitals for many decades. It allows for honest encounter between children, their families, and their care providers, for the intersubjective and interpersonal encounters which form the basis of who we are.

***

In the end, taking a childist perspective on the participation of children in medical decision-making at the end of life means confronting the fact that our cultural and institutional structures are biased against including children through their structures, goals, accounts of rationality, and definitions of meaningful participation. In order for the rights of children to participate, enshrined in policy, to be made practice, we need to embark upon a childist reconstruction of our cultural and institutional spaces that puts the participation of children first.

The questions of decision-making in this chapter have, in effect, driven this entire project. Thinking deeply about children's participation in end-of-life decision-making has compelled me to step back and consider who a child is, what death is, how we understand children's moral agency, and how we think about choice. Most of all, it has shown that to properly address the issues facing children with life-limiting illness, we must be willing to put aside our preconceptions and to talk to children, to ask them questions, to speak honestly with them, to recognize their gifts and abilities, and to see them as having something to teach us.

Childhood is biologically determined but also culturally constructed; we can and should challenge visions of childhood that are at odds with what it means to be intersubjective subjects and children of God. Childhood is not simply an unchanging and monolithic reality: instead, it includes fetuses, babies, toddlers, and children, and bleeds into the lives of tweens, teenagers, adolescents, youths, and young adults, adults, and the elderly. We have much to learn from the ways in which childhood has been understood in different time periods and across different cultures, not as ideals to return to, but as tools to evaluate both cultural and theological conceptions of childhood that do not align with what it means to be a child in light of the Christian gospel, a gospel in which we are told that the Incarnate Son of God became a child, and in which children are lifted up as models of discipleship. Childhood is not simply a state we leave behind, a mere stopping point on the journey to full humanity. Instead, children are already fully human, and childhood extends into the eschaton, as we become ever more aware of our dependency on divine love. Recognizing the gifts of childhood, and what children have to teach us about what it means to be human, requires an exercise in humility.

It also requires courage: We must be willing to face our own inadequacies and fears, especially our fear of death. An ethical restructuring of moral agency in light of what children reveal asks us to put aside our own pretensions toward independence and autonomy; it means acknowledging that we have moral limitations. We cannot simply do what we like. This account of moral agency is based on understanding children as intersubjective and self-transcendent subjects. Intersubjectivity supposes a relationality internal to our subjectivity and constitutive of it. This account of intersubjectivity also allows us to posit an asymmetry of relationship between adult and child that is predicated on a common humanity—both in the obligations adults have toward children, and the ways in which the goods of childhood call adults to see the world in new ways. This account of self-transcendence, and its recognition of a wider notion of rationality, allows us to recognize that children look and listen, they experience and observe, and they reflect, ask questions, posit answers, make judgments, and act; they are curious and they use their imagination. In other words, children are already moral agents.

Because children are subjects and moral agents, they are capable of creating meaning in the dying process, and capable of participating in making meaningful decisions with respect to their end-of-life care. Both decision-making and meaning-making at the end of life should be viewed as shared ventures between children and adults, where each brings their own particular strengths and gifts. In this way, the final acts of caring for children with life-limiting illness are not viewed as a binary between what a child can do for himself or what is done for or to him, but rather a joint venture.

In this joint venture, we can learn from children. What are difficult tasks—attending to the question of dying children, taking seriously their suffering, and acknowledging the ways in which we as a society have failed to care for them—can also be rewarding ones, in which children, sharing in this properly joint venture, reveal to us what it means to be human, which is to be children of God. The tragedy and sorrow of a child's death also remind us that completion and meaning are ultimately found, not in our choices at the end of life, but in God. Our structures can never overcome the grief and feelings of senselessness and hopelessness we experience when caring for dying children. We should fight to meet their needs as best we can, but also acknowledge that there are limits to our efforts. Children remind us that none of us have full control. We have no answers to why children die or why they suffer, but we can learn from their endless capacity to create and communicate meaning where we thought it impossible. We can find hope in the knowledge that they are already living the goal of human life. Sharing with children in the task of dying well means that together we can learn how to befriend death.

NOTES

1 J. R. R. Tolkien, *The Two Towers* (London: HarperCollins, 2002), 32.
2 Imelda Coyne, "Consultation with Children in Hospital: Children, Parents' and Nurses' Perspectives," in *Journal of Clinical Nursing* 15 (2006) 61–71; Imelda Coyne, "Response," *Journal of Clinical Nursing* 15 (2006), 794; Jeremy Jolley, "Commentary on Coyne I (2006) 'Consultation with Children in Hospital: Children, Parents' and Nurses' Perspectives'," *Journal of Clinical Nursing* 15 (2006) 61–71, 791–793.
3 See summary in Vida Jeremic, et al., "Participation of Children in Medical Decision-Making: Challenges and Potential Solutions," in *Bioethical Inquiry* 13 (2016): 525–534.
4 Penny Lawrence, "Hearing and Acting with the Voices of Children in Early Childhood," in *Journal of the British Academy* 8 (2022): 79.
5 Jolley, "Commentary," 792.
6 Jody L. Lin, et al., "Parent Perspectives in Shared Decision-Making for Children with Medical Complexity," in *Academic Pediatrics* 20 (2020): 1106; Kirk D. Wyatt, et al., "Shared Decision Making in Pediatrics: A Systematic Review and Meta-analysis," *Academic Pediatrics* 15 (2015): 577.
7 Lin, et al., "Parent Perspectives," 1106.
8 Coyne, "Consultation," 61–71; Cristina Nova, et al., "The Physician–Patient–Parent Communication: A Qualitative Perspective on the Child's Contribution," in *Patient Education and Counseling* 58 (2005): 327–333; Imelda Coyne and Lisa Kirwan, "Ascertaining Children's Wishes and Feelings about Hospital Life," *Journal of Child Health Care* 16 (2012): 293–304; see also Ellen A. Lipstein, et al., "An Emerging Field of Research: Challenges in Pediatric Decision Making," in *Medical Decision Making* (2015): 403–408; Francine Buchanan, et al., "What makes difficult decisions so difficult?: An activity theory analysis of decision making for physicians treating children with medical complexity," in *Patient Education and Counseling* 103 (2020): 2260–2268.
9 Michael Wyness, "Children's Participation: Definitions, Narratives and Disputes" in *Theorising Childhood: Citizenship, Rights, and Participation*, eds. Claudio Baraldi and Tom Cockburn (London: Palgrave MacMillan, 2018), 57.

10 Jolley, "Commentary," 792.

11 See, among others, Jolley, "Commentary," 791–793; Coyne, "Consultation," 61–71; Hoffmaster, "The Rationality and Morality of Dying Children," in *The Hastings Center Report* 41 (2011): 30–42; Myra Bluebond-Langner, et al., "Preferred place of death for children and young people with life-limiting and life-threatening conditions: A systematic review of the literature and recommendations for future inquiry and policy," in *Palliative Medicine* 27 (2013): 711; Katharina M. Ruhe, et al., "Rational Capacity: Broadening the Notion of Decision-Making Capacity in Paediatric Healthcare," in *Bioethical Inquiry* 13 (2016): 515–516.

12 Hoffmaster, "Rationality and Morality," 31.

13 Buchanan, "What Makes Difficult Decisions So Difficult," 2260; see also Wyatt, et al., "Shared Decision Making"; Lin, et al., "Parent Perspectives."

14 Jeremic, et al., "Participation," 527.

15 Izetta Smith, "Preschool Children 'Play' out Their Grief," in *Death Studies* 15 (1991): 169–176.

16 Wyatt, et al., "Shared Decision Making," 577–578.

17 Wyness, "Children's Participation," 57.

18 See, for example, Thomas Reynolds, *Vulnerable Communion: A Theology of Disability and Hospitality* (Grand Rapids: Brazos Press, 2008).

19 Jolley, "Commentary," 793.

20 Lipstein, et al., "An Emerging Field of Research," 403.

21 Margaret Urban Walker, *Moral Understandings: A Feminist Study in Ethics,* 2nd ed. (Oxford: Oxford University Press, 2007), 7–8.

22 Lipstein, et al., "An Emerging Field of Research," 405.

23 There are many related and larger deficiencies in the way medicine deals with personhood, and how it envisions the human being and the goods of medicine. Studies that address these larger issues, including the seductive power of medicine, the denuded goods or aims, and the vision of the human person, include Jeffrey P. Bishop *The Anticipatory Corpse* (2011), Nicanor Pier Giorgio Austriaco *Biomedicine and Beatitude* (2012), Joel Shuman and Brian Volck *Reclaiming the Body* (2006), Carl Elliot *Better Than Well* (2004), and Stanley Hauerwas *Suffering Presence* (1986).

24 Tom L. Beauchamp and James F. Childress, *Principles of Biomedical Ethics*, 4th ed. (New York: Oxford University Press, 1994). See also Jaclyn Duffin, *History of Medicine: A Scandalously Short Introduction*, 2nd ed. (Toronto: University of Toronto Press, 2010); John H. Evans, *Playing God?: Human Genetic Engineering and the Rationalization of Public Bioethical Discourse* (Chicago: University of Chicago Press, 2002).

25 Hoffmaster, "Rationality and Morality," 30.

26 Brian S. Carter, Marcia Levetown and Sarah E. Friebert, eds, *Palliative Care for Infants, Children, and Adolescents: A Practical Handbook*, 2nd ed. (Baltimore: Johns Hopkins University Press, 2011), 26.

27 Cf. Julius Kovesi, *Moral Notions* (London: Rutledge, 1971); G. E. M. Anscombe, "Under a Description" in *Noûs* 13 (1979): 219–233.

28 Hoffmaster, "Rationality and Morality," 32.

29 Chris Feudtner, et al., "Surrogate's Personal Sense of Duty as a Crucial Element in Medical Decision Making: Ethical, Empirical, and Experience-Based Perspectives,"

in *The Ethics of Shared Decision Making*, ed. John Lantos (Oxford: Oxford University Press, 2021), 11.

30 Jeremic, et al., "Participation," 527.

31 Jeremic, et al., "Participation," 527.

32 Jeremic, et al., "Participation," 527.

33 Mary Ann McCabe, "Involving Children and Adolescents in Medical Decision Making: Developmental and Clinical Considerations," in *Journal of Pediatric Psychology* 21.4 (1996): 507.

34 Jeremic, et al., "Participation," 526.

35 Childress and Beauchamp, *Principles*, 58; Childress and Beauchamp also admit in the chapter that basically no one is autonomous for all things even at their peak. So this calls into question why something that almost no one achieves is the basis for an entire ethical system!

36 Luc Bovens, "Child Euthanasia: Should we just not talk about it?" in *Journal of Medical Ethics* 41 (2015): 630.

37 Jeremic, et al., "Participation," 525.

38 Michelle M. Ernst, Carrie Piazza-Waggoner, and Heather Ciesielski, "The Role of Paediatric Psychologists in Facilitating Medical Decision Making in the Care of Critically Ill Young Children," in *Clinical Practice in Pediatric Psychology* 3 (2015): 120–121.

39 Ruhe, et al., "Rational Capacity," 515.

40 As implied in mature minor frameworks. See, for example, Carey DeMichaelis, Randi Zlotnik Shaul, and Adam Rapoport, "Medical Assistance in Dying at a Paediatric hospital" in *Journal of Medical Ethics* 45 (2019): 60–67.

41 Robert M. Doran, *Theology and the Dialectics of History* (Toronto: University of Toronto Press, 2001), 573–575.

42 Myra Bluebond-Langner, *The Private Worlds of Dying Children* (Princeton: Princeton University Press, 1980), 189–197.

43 Hoffmaster, "Rationality and Morality," 31.

44 Doran, *Theology*, 576.

45 In this way, this model for shared decision-making, because it is grounded in an account of the human person as intersubjective subject who aims for the true and the good, helps explain why agreement between parents and children has moral validity, a concern raised by Giles Birchley about standard models of shared decision-making, which are procedural accounts not grounded in an account of the human person and the aims and goods of what it means to be human. Cf. Giles Birchley, "Deciding Together? Best Interests and Shared Decision-Making in Paediatric Intensive Care" in *Health Care Analysis* 22 (2014): 203–222.

46 Ruhe, et al., "Relational Capacity," 520–521.

47 Lin, et al., "Parent Perspectives," 1103.

48 Lin, et al., "Parent Perspectives," 1103.

49 Feudtner, et al., "Surrogate's Personal Sense of Duty," 11.

50 Christine Harrison, "Truth Telling in Pediatrics: What They Don't Know Might Hurt Them," in *Pediatric Bioethics*, ed. Geoffrey Miller (Cambridge: Cambridge University Press, 2010), 73–4; United Nations General Assembly, *Convention on the Rights of the Child*. United Nations (1989).

51 George MacDonald, *At the Back of the North Wind* (London: Alfred A. Knoff, 2001), 203–213.

52 Beauchamp and Childress, *Principles*, 58.
53 Feudtner, et al., "Surrogate's Personal Sense of Duty," 15.
54 Feudtner, et al., "Surrogate's Personal Sense of Duty," 21.
55 Bluebond-Langner, *Private Worlds*, 7.
56 Wyatt, et al., "Shared Decision Making," 578.
57 Laura Armstrong, "SickKids: Shared Decision Making Helps with the Life's Weighty Issues" *Toronto Star*. 7 May 2015. https://tinyurl.com/5n926tw5
58 McCabe, "Involving Children," 506.
59 Jo-Eileen Guylay, *The Dying Child* (Toronto: McGraw-Hill, 1978), 10.
60 Guylay, *Dying Child*, 11.

Epilogue
The Good Death?

A discussion of decision-making at the end of life cannot avoid the question of child euthanasia. Enthusiasm for child euthanasia is gaining traction in many parts of the Western world, as traditional arguments regarding the intrinsic evil of the practice are no longer convincing to many. Arguments in favor of euthanasia rely on two poorly defined but rhetorically and emotionally powerful concepts: autonomy and unbearable suffering. Less explicit, but perhaps equally powerful, are underlying cultural conceptions of the good death and the attendant assumption that death and dying are meaningless. In this epilogue, I want to consider the question of child euthanasia in light of the account of children and their ethical intentionality laid out in this book. To lay my cards on the table, I argue that reconfiguring our account of the moral life to include children undermines the foundation on which arguments for (and some against) euthanasia are predicated.

So far, child euthanasia is legal in only two countries, Belgium and the Netherlands, and proponents are pushing to extend Canadian legislation to minors.[1] Euthanasia means the active ending of someone's life, usually by a physician, usually on account of life-limiting illness or disability. It differs from physician-assisted suicide, where patients are supplied with a lethal substance but administer it themselves. While I will speak specifically about euthanasia, most of what I have to say applies equally to physician-assisted suicide, since I am not considering issues of physicians' right to refuse and other ethical decisions along those lines, but rather underlying autonomy-based arguments in favor of the practice of actively choosing death. Euthanasia differs from allowing a patient to die through cessation of treatment. As a moral category, however, euthanasia is not limited to a certain medical procedure, but includes all active forms of ending someone's life, such that any treatment decision undertaken for the purpose of ending life would be included.

It is difficult to give a detailed account of scholarly arguments for pediatric euthanasia because there are few such arguments made.[2] This is primarily because, as with most difficult questions of pediatric medical ethics, existing scholarship views the discussions around adult euthanasia as sufficient for its purposes and only considers what adjustments need to be made for a pediatric setting. Thus, pediatric arguments simply apply the discussion of euthanasia for adults to children, either by advocating for a capacity approach in which the children are mature minors and therefore in the same ethical category as adults, or by assuming the right of parents or guardians to decide, on the basis of surrogate autonomy.[3] For example, the arguments in favor of including minors in an expansion of Canada's euthanasia laws refer to including young people in the definition of "capable adult."[4] In this case, the general assumption seems to be that euthanasia is not different than any other decision at the end of life, and so existing metrics for making capability assessments should apply.

Proponents of euthanasia for both children and adults cite autonomy—a person's right to make their own decisions free from restraint, on the basis that the individual is the final legislator of right and wrong—and the "unbearable" suffering which can accompany dying as the two major reasons that justify actively seeking death. In Luc Bovens's summary of arguments against euthanasia for minors in Belgium, it is clear that the arguments in favor of euthanasia primarily rely on the cessation of suffering, as many responses to these arguments argue that there are many ways to end the suffering of minors without prematurely ending their lives. Most of the objections to the practice raised in the Belgian context have to do with autonomy, specifically the lack of autonomy, whether in the context of a minor's lack of capacity for discernment or the increased risk of coercion.[5] In their paper on medical assistance in dying (MAID) for mature minors, DeMichelis, et al., list the two purposes of euthanasia as "alleviat[ing] unendurable suffering and facilitat[ing] the patient dying on their own terms."[6] Arguments in favor of euthanasia for infants are usually predicated on ending suffering, though these arguments rely on a notion of parental surrogate autonomy—that is, on the idea that the best interests of the child are those of the parents.[7] Discussions in a *Pediatrics* Ethics Round about laws in the Netherlands cite both suffering and the right to "self-determination" as reasons for legalizing euthanasia, and the Dutch minister who announced the expansion of laws to children between one and twelve expressed it as important for children who are "suffering hopelessly and unbearably."[8]

There are two other issues that undergird arguments in favor of euthanasia. First, as I described in chapter 3, the cultural ideal regarding the good death is characterized by conscious choice and by control. That is, to borrow DeMichelis's words, we should get to die on our own terms. This view finds death and dying inherently meaningless, because meaning is only derived from conscious, rational choice. If euthanasia is, as DeMichelis, et al. describe it, about facilitating death on the patient's terms, we must be cognizant that cultural ideals around death dictate these terms; in the case of children, these ideals dictate the terms of their parents and caregivers. Second, arguments in favor of euthanasia stem from a consequentialist approach to ethics, which sees euthanasia as not meaningfully distinct from other medical practices, like the withdrawal of treatment, but understands it to be practically and ethically equivalent to other treatments at the end of life. These issues are not often acknowledged. Given the deficiencies in pediatric bioethics I highlighted in the previous chapter, it is troubling that the models for consultation with respect to MAID and mature minors in Canada do not include ethicists in the list of those who should be consulted on the topic.[9]

Those who think euthanasia and physician-assisted suicide are wrong writ large, on the grounds of traditional beliefs about the intrinsic evil of the practice, or more recent arguments against such prioritization of autonomy from feminist or disability perspectives, will also hold that it is wrong for children.[10] My own argument against the practice tends in the other direction. It is the consideration of *children* and what it means for them to share in the human moral life that undermines arguments in favor of euthanasia, for both children and for adults. The view of children for which I have argued in this project—children as intersubjective and self-transcendent subjects, as moral agents and sharers in the same humanity as adults—has required a reassessment of the moral life, undermining the foundation of autonomy on which arguments in favor of euthanasia rest. To include children as moral agents compels us to change how we understand moral agency and personhood, which in turn undermines the liberal, individualistic, autonomous premises of arguments for euthanasia.

To put it another way, the childist account of ethical intentionality put forward in this book, which is an account of not only how children engage in the moral world, but also what their moral agency and subjectivity reveal about *human* morality, offers an (often contradictory) account of human relationality, rationality, language, and goals of life that is much different than the story of autonomy. Whether in considering constitutive versus enframing philosophies of language, the account of narrow formal reason versus a creative, imitative, received reason, or the goal of rational control versus childhood in God, taking children seriously reveals that the moral life of human beings is fundamentally different than that imagined by theories of autonomy and self-determination. Any autonomy we have is creaturely and relational: It is always a response to received morality and lived out in a shared, intersubjective way. That is, we do not have the right to determine the manner of our death. We do not have control over life and death. Moreover, instead of accepting a (faulty) adult-oriented vision of death and expanding it to children, we should remember that the goal of Christian discipleship is to be a child of God: *We should all die as children.*

But what of suffering? While moral arguments in favor of euthanasia come back, ultimately, to the idea that we ought to have control over the manner of our death, more compelling to many is the suffering at the end of life. A poignant argument in favor of euthanasia is the idea that children who are dying are suffering and that we have an ethical obligation to end this intolerable or irremediable suffering, described by words like "unendurable" and "hopeless."

But children rarely speak of their condition as hopeless or describe their experience as one of unbearable suffering. Their verbal and nonverbal expressions may communicate extensive suffering, but these experiences are interpreted by those who care for them according to their own frameworks.[11] Who, then, is allowed to identify intolerable suffering? It is interpreted according to adults. While in a properly shared venture, interpretation is entirely appropriate, it is also always open to bias. Moreover, as I explained in the third chapter, we need to challenge the idea that suffering is inherently meaningless because meaning is tied up in adult notions of rational, individualized capacity. Further, the nebulous issue of suffering loses much of its moral weight when we turn to addressing specific sources of suffering.[12] Until we do all we can to address those sources of suffering, it is hard to see how the harm of death could be outweighed by an external judgment regarding the quality of a child's life.

Given the research into all the ways we fail to engage with children, to properly attend to and treat their pain, and to combat their isolation and fear, and especially given the ways in which children feel guilty about the burden of their illness on their parents, and deeply desire to comfort those they love, we ought first to fully address these factors before declaring that the only option for a child is termination of her life. When the suffering of children is described as hopeless, we should ask ourselves: From where do children get their hope? In what is their hope? What enables any of us to endure suffering? I argued in chapter 3 that children can and do find meaning in death and dying, and we can both learn from them, and help them to create meaning. A dying child's community plays a significant role in determining whether the child experiences her situation as hopeless, or whether she sees her suffering as meaningful. There is much we can do to comfort children by helping them to find hope and meaning at the end of their lives. We have the opportunity to partner with children in all areas of life and inquiry, in what I have described as a shared venture. When we see dying not as an alien and other realm, but as a life task, then we can see that it is one more opportunity for a joint venture.

Throughout this book, I have talked about attending to children, to all that they reveal about life, to all that they have to teach us, to all that they reveal about our obligations toward them, and to their suffering. This last one will always be the most difficult. Simone Weil writes, "To give one's attention to the suffering of others . . . involves sacrifice."[13] It means being willing to face the fact that we cannot control many of life's circumstances, that we cannot control life and death. Christians want to avoid child suffering not only because we do not want our children to suffer, but because facing their suffering can and will change our faith. We worry that we might lose our faith in the face of these unanswerable questions of why this child and why this disease. We worry because there are no easy lessons for moral improvement or trite ideas about God's purpose in such circumstances. Dying children scare adults. But instead of turning away, we must be willing to walk the dark road, to question our assumptions about the good life and the good death, to think deeply about who children are, what we owe them, and what they are capable of. We need to recognize them as moral agents, intersubjective and self-transcending subjects, and beloved children of God.

However, I hesitate to end this book simply with a moral injunction against euthanasia. After all, what is interesting and important is not so much what we cannot do, but *why* we should not do it, and most importantly, *what we should do instead*. As I have suggested throughout the book, there is so much that we *can* do, and so many ways that we can and should turn our efforts as much to making a peaceful and meaningful death possible as to delaying death and curing diseases. Instead of seeking a quick fix for suffering, we should turn our attention to eradicating situations in which desires for euthanasia arise. This means creating a society in which we attend to who children are, welcome them, and create space for their families and caregivers.

Children are not merely passive receptacles of care but have active vocations of revealing God to the world, whether they live for an hour or for years. Children show us how to welcome God by calling us to compassion and by modeling discipleship. From children, we can learn how to put aside our pretense of self-sufficiency and free ourselves to acknowledge both our own pain and that of others. Children help us to learn what it means to live without being in control, instead of making control the criteria of human flourishing. Thus, a dying child is not excluded from God's purposes but rather is part of his ministry. Dying children fulfill the purposes of God by teaching us to face our own death, and by showing us how to enter our second childhood with faith and obedience. We must be cautious, though, about how we interpret their vocation. God does not make children ill in order to teach us lessons. The death of a child is not somehow made valuable or worthwhile by the fact that it can teach us about God and ourselves. Instead, a child's value comes from her shared relationship with others in God.

God is already at work in the life of a child, and we should be also. This means that we should neither deny nor idealize the suffering of children but encounter it with honesty and compassion. We must take the time to be present with children, to listen to them, to ask them questions, to pay attention to the myriad of ways in which they communicate that may seem foreign or strange to us, and to give them a chance to participate in their own care, even if it is a challenge to include them or makes things take a longer time than we would like. We should also pay attention to the types of stories to which children are drawn; if we are tempted to act according to a narrow account of rationality, of the moral life, and of reality, the fantastical provides a remedy, reminding us of the plurality of meaning and the possibilities found in every person if only we are willing to put aside our narrow ways and see them. From children, we can learn about the strange and sometimes wonderful possibilities of the world at the North Wind's back.

Helping people to deal with the senselessness of child death, to make meaning together in the dying process, and to welcome grieving families requires not only a transformation of our medical institutions, but a transformation of our culture. It means becoming people who are willing to face our mortality, to grieve, to resist the flight from suffering. That is, we should be a society in which we work together to befriend death. Moreover, as those who know the gospel, we cannot support the cultural conspiracy of silence around death and engage in the charade that we will all live forever. Instead, we must openly and bravely acknowledge that we will all die, and thus be willing to witness and comfort those who are dying. We can do this because we know that our death and dying is part of a larger story. In the death and resurrection of Jesus, we are now all able to participate in the life of God for all eternity; in the world at North Wind's back, we will all live as children of God.

NOTES

1 Brouwer, et al., "Should Pediatric Euthanasia be Legalized?" in *Pediatrics* 141 (2018): 1.

2 The topic is not discussed in Geoffrey Miller, ed., *Pediatric Bioethics* (Cambridge: Cambridge University Press, 2010); Brian S. Carter, Marcia Levetown and Sarah E. Friebert, eds., *Palliative Care for Infants, Children, and Adolescents: A Practical Handbook*, 2nd ed. (Baltimore: Johns Hopkins University Press, 2011); Rita Pfund and Susan Fowler-Kerry, eds., *Perspectives on Palliative Care for Children and Young People: A Global Discourse*. New York: Radcliffe Publishing, 2010.

3 See Luc Bovens, "Child Euthanasia: Should We Just Not Talk about It?" in *Journal of Medical Ethics* 41 (2015): 630–634; Carey DeMichelis, Randi Zlotnik Shaul, and Adam Rapoport, "Medical Assistance in Dying at a Paediatric Hospital" *Journal of Medical Ethics* 45 (2019): 61; Eduard Vergahen and Pieter J. J. Sauer, "The Groningen Protocol—Euthanasia for Severely Ill Newborns," in *New England Journal of Medicine* 352 (2005): 959–962.

4 DeMichelis, et al., "Medical Assistance," 60–62.

5 Bovens, "Child Euthanasia," 630–634. In the Belgian context, as he explains, the legislation applies to children deemed capable of making their own medical decisions.

6 DeMichelis, et al., "Medical Assistance," 60–62.

7 See, for example, Verhagen and Sauer, "The Groningen Protocol," 959–962.

8 Brouwer, et al., "Pediatric Euthanasia," 4; BBC News "Netherlands Backs Euthanasia for Terminally Ill Children under-12" October 14, 2020, https://www.bbc.com/news/world-europe-54538288

9 Illustrated, for example, in DeMichelis, et al., "Medical Assistance," 61; See also Dawn Davies, "Medical Assistance in Dying: A Paediatric Perspective," *Paediatrics & Child Health* (2018): 125–130.

10 See, for example, S. Callahan, "A Feminist Case against Euthanasia: Women Should be Especially Wary of Arguments for 'the Freedom to Die,'" in *Health Progress* 77 (1996):

21–29; Tim Stainton, "Disability, Vulnerability and Assisted Death: Commentary on Tuffrey-Wijne, Curfs, Finlay and Hollins," in *BMC Medical Ethics* 20 (2019): 1–6; Nigel Biggar, *Aiming to Kill: The Ethics of Suicide and Euthanasia* (London: Darton Longman & Todd, 2004).

11 Dr. Miriam Vos, quoted in Michael Cook, "Dutch Pediatricians Seek Child Euthanasia," in *National Right to Life News*, (2016): 42. This is made more serious by the fact that assessments of the child for anxiety or depression is rarely done. Hinds, et al., "Key Factors," 72.

12 Harvey Chochinov, et al., "Desire for Death in the Terminally Ill," in *American Journal of Psychiatry* 152 (1995): 1185–1191.

13 Quoted in Stuart Jesson, "Simone Weil: Suffering, Attention and Compassionate Thought," in *Studies in Christian Ethics* 27 (2014): 190.

Bibliography

Aasgaard, Reidar. "Paul as a Child: Children and Childhood in the Letters of the Apostle." *Journal of Biblical Literature* 126, no. 1 (2007): 129–59.

Adams, Harry. *Justice for Children: Autonomy Development and the State.* Albany: State University of New York Press, 2007.

Akard, Terrah Foster, and Mary Jo Gilmer. "Invisible Communities of Dying Children and Their Loved Ones." *Palliative and Supportive Care* 13 (2015): 1501–1503.

Alexandre-Bidon, Danièle and Dider Lett. *Les Enfants au Moyen Age: Ve-XVe siècles.* Hachette Littératures, 1997.

André, Nicolas, Jean Gaudart, Jean Bernard, and B. Chabrol. "Quelle place pour l'enfant dans la prise de décision en pédiatrie?" *Archies de Pédiatrie* 12, (2005): 1068–1074.

Anscombe, G. E. M. *Faith in a Hard Ground: Essays on Religion, Philosophy and Ethics by G. E. M. Anscombe.* Edited by Mary Geach and Luke Gormally. Exeter: Imprint Academic, 2008.

———. *Human Life, Action and Ethics: Essays by G. E. M. Anscombe.* Edited by Mary Geach and Luke Gormally. Exeter: Imprint Academic, 2005.

———. "Under a Description," *Noûs* 13 (1979): 219–233.

Ariès, Philippe. *Centuries of Childhood: A Social History of Family Life.* Translated by Robert Baldick. New York: Vintage, 1962.

Arman, Maria, and Arne Rehnsfeldt. "The 'Little Extra' that Alleviates Suffering." *Nursing Ethics* 14, no. 3 (2007): 373–386.

Arman, Maria, and Arne Rehnsfeldt. "The Presence of Love in Ethical Caring." *Nursing Forum* 41, no. 1 (2006): 4–12.

Armstrong, Laura. "SickKids: Shared Decision Making Helps with the Life's Weighty Issues." *Toronto Star*, May 7, 2015. https://tinyurl.com/5n926tw5

Augustine, Saint, Sister Mary Sarah Muldowney, Harold B. Jaffee, Sister Mary Francis McDonald, Sister Luanne Meagher, Sister M. Clement Eagan, and Mary E. DeFerrari. "Against Lying." In *Treatises on Various Subjects (The Fathers of the Church, Volume 16)*, translated by Roy J. Deferrari, 113–179. Washington, DC: Catholic University of American Press, 1952.

Avci, Keziban, Songül Çinaroglu, and Mehmet Top. "Perceptions of Pediatric Nurses on Ethical Decision Making Processes." *Systemic Practice and Action Research* 30, no. 1 (2017): 67–84.

von Baeyer, C. L., L. Uman, C.T. Chambers, and A. Gouthro. "Can We Screen Young Children for Their Ability to Provide Accurate Self-Reports of Pain?" *Pain* 152 (2011): 1327–1333.

Bagatell, Rochelle, Robyn Meyer, Sandra Herron, Alice Berger, and Rodrigo Villar. "When Children Die: A Seminar Series for Pediatric Residents." *Pediatrics* 110, no. 2 (2002): 348–353.

Bahler, Brock. *Childlike Peace in Merleau-Ponty and Levinas: Intersubjectivity as Dialectical Spiral*. New York: Lexington Books, 2016.

Baker, Jen. "Traditions and Anxieties of (Un)timely Traditions in *Jude the Obscure*." *The Thomas Hardy Journal* 33, (2017): 61–84.

Bakke, O. M. *When Children Became People: The Birth of Childhood in Early Christianity*. Minneapolis: Fortress Press, 2005.

von Balthasar, Hans Urs. *Unless You Become Like This Child*. Translated by Erasmo Leiva-Merikakis. San Francisco: Ignatius Press, 1991.

Banner, Michael. *The Ethics of Everyday Life: Moral Theology, Social Anthropology, and the Imagination of the Human*. Oxford: Oxford University Press, 2014.

Baraldi, Claudio and Tom Cockburn, eds. *Theorising Childhood: Citizenship, Rights and Participation*. London: Palgrave MacMillan, 2018.

Barina, Rachelle, and Jeffrey P. Bishop. "Maturing the Minor, Marginalizing the Family: On the Social Construction of the Mature Minor." *Journal of Medicine and Philosophy* 38, no. 3 (2013): 300–314.

Bartholdson, Cecilia, Kim Lützén, Klas Blomgren, and Pernilla Pergert. "Experiences of Ethical Issues When Caring for Children with Cancer." *Cancer Nursing* 38, no. 2 (2015): 125–132.

Baumann, Holger. "Reconsidering Relational Autonomy. Personal Autonomy for Socially Embedded and Temporally Extended Selves." *Analyse & Kritik* 30, no. 2 (2008): 445–468.

Beale, Estela A., Walter F. Baile, and Joann Aaron. "Silence Is Not Golden: Communicating With Children Dying From Cancer." *Journal of Clinical Oncology* 23, no. 15 (2005): 3629–3631.

Beauchamp, Tom L., James F. Childress. *Principles of Biomedical Ethics*, 4th ed. New York: Oxford University Press, 1994.

Bell, Nancy. "Ethics in Child Research: Rights, Reason and Responsibilities." *Children's Geographies* 6, no. 1 (2008): 7–20.

Benini, Franca, Roberta Vecchi, and Marcello Orzalesi. "A Charter for the Rights of the Dying Child." Correspondence, *The Lancet* 383 (2014): 1547–1548.

Berg, Siri F., Odd G. Paulsen, and Brian S. Carter. "Why Were They in Such a Hurry to See Her Die?" *American Journal of Hospice & Palliative Medicine* 30, no. 4 (2012): 406–408.

Berglund, Catherine, and John Devereux. "Consent to Medical Treatment: Children Making Medical Decisions for Others." *Australian Journal of Forensic Science* 32, no. 1 (2000): 25–36.

Berryman, Jerome W. *Children and the Theologians: Clearing the Way for Grace*. New York: Morehouse, 2009.

Bhroin, M. N. "'A Slice of Life': The Interrelationships among Art, Play and the 'Real' Life of the Young Child." *International Journal of Education & the Arts* 8, no.16 (2007): 1–24.

Biggar, Nigel. *Aiming to Kill: The Ethics of Suicide and Euthanasia*. London: Darton Longman & Todd, 2004.

Billone, Amy. "Hovering between Irony and Innocence: George MacDonald's 'The Light Princess' and the Gravity of Childhood." *Mosaic: A Journal for the Interdisciplinary Study of Literature* 37, no. 1 (2004): 1–10.

Birchley, Giles, Rachael Gooberman-Hill, Zuzana Deans, James Fraser, and Richard Huxtable. "'Best Interests' in Paediatric Intensive Care: An Empirical Ethics Study." *Archives Disease in Childhood* 102 (2017): 930–935.

Birchley, Giles. "Deciding Together? Best Interests and Shared Decision-Making in Paediatric Intensive Care." *Health Care Analysis* 22 (2014): 203–222.

Bishop, Jeffrey P. *The Anticipatory Corpse: Medicine, Power, and the Care of the Dying*. Notre Dame: University of Notre Dame Press, 2011.

Bloom, Paul. *Just Babies: The Origins of Good and Evil*. New York: Random House, 2013.

Bluebond-Langner, Myra, Emma Beecham, Bridget Candy, Richard Langner, and Louise Jones. "Preferred Place of Death for Children and Young People with Life-Limiting and Life-Threatening Conditions: A Systematic Review of the Literature and Recommendations for Future Inquiry and Policy." *Palliative Medicine* 27 (2013): 705–713.

———. *The Private Worlds of Dying Children.* Princeton: Princeton University Press, 1980.

Bonoti, Fotini, Angeliki Leondari, and Adelais Mastora. "Exploring Children's Understanding of Death: Through Drawings and the Death Concept Questionnaire." *Death Studies* 37, no. 1 (2013): 47–60.

Bornstein, Marc H. "Cultural Approaches to Parenting." *Parent Sci Pract* 12, no. 2–3 (2013): 1–10.

Bovens, Luc. "Child Euthanasia: Should We Just Not Talk about It?" *Journal of Medical Ethics* 41 (2015): 630–634.

Brennan, Patrick McKinley, ed. *The Vocation of the Child.* Grand Rapids: Eerdmans, 2008.

Brierly, Joe, Jim Linthicum, and Andy Petros. "Should Religious Beliefs Be Allowed to Stonewall a Secular Approach to Withdrawing and Withholding Treatment in Children?" *Journal of Medical Ethics* 39 (2013): 573–577.

Brock, Dan W., and Allen E. Buchanan. *Deciding for Others: The Ethics of Surrogate Decision Making.* New York: Cambridge University Press, 1989.

Brody, Hugh. "'The Deepest Silences': What Lies behind the Arctic's Indigenous Suicide Crisis." *The Guardian*, July 21, 2022. https://tinyurl.com/2dk92rvn

Brouwer, Marije, Christopher Kaczor, Margaret P. Battin, Els Maeckelberghe, John D. Lantos, and Eduard Verhagen. "Should Pediatric Euthanasia be Legalized?" *Pediatrics* 141, no. 2 (2018): 1–5.

Bubel, Katharine. "Knowing God 'Other-wise': The Wise Old Woman Archetype in George MacDonald's The Princess and The Goblin, The Princess and Curdie and 'The Golden Key'." North Wind: A *Journal of George MacDonald Studies* 25, no. 1 (2006): 1–8.

Buchanan, Francine, Claudia Lai, Eyal Cohen, Golda Milo-Manson, Aviv Shachak. "Decision-Making for Parents of Children with Medical Complexities: Activity Theory Analysis." *Journal of Participatory Medicine* 14, no. 1 (2022): 1–12.

Buchanan, Francine, Eyal Cohen, Golda Milo-Manson, Aviv Shachak. "What Makes Difficult Decisions So Difficult?: An Activity Theory Analysis of Decision Making for Physicians Treating Children with Medical Complexity." *Patient Education and Counseling* 103, no. 11 (2020): 2260–2268.

Bunge, Marcia J., ed. *The Child in the Bible.* Grand Rapids: Eerdmans, 2008.

———, ed. *The Child in Christian Thought.* Grand Rapids: Eerdmans, 2001.

Burke, Tony. "Depictions of Children in the Apocryphal Infancy Gospels." *Studies in Religion/Sciences Religieuses* 41, no. 3 (2012): 388–400.

Burman, Erica. *Deconstructing Developmental Psychology.* 3rd ed. London: Routledge, 2017.

Burns, Kevin J. "Modern Medicine, Theory and Practice." Review of *The Anticipatory Corpse: Medicine, Power, and the Care of the Dying,* by Jefferey P. Bishop. Perspectives on Political Science, October–December 2015.

Burt, Michael. "Phantastes and the Development of the Imagination," *North Wind* 35 (2016): 89–103.

Byrne, Patrick H. *The Ethics of Discernment: Lonergan's Foundations for Ethics.* Toronto: University of Toronto Press, 2016.

Callahan, S. "A Feminist Case against Euthanasia. Women Should Be Especially Wary of Arguments for 'the Freedom to Die'." *Health Progress* 77, no. 6 (1996): 21–29.

Carter, Brian S. "Why Palliative Care for Children is Preferable to Euthanasia." *American Journal of Hospital & Palliative Care* 33 (2016): 1–3.

Carter, Brian S., Marcia Levetown and Sarah E. Friebert, eds. *Palliative Care for Infants, Children, and Adolescents: A Practical Handbook.* 2nd ed. Baltimore: Johns Hopkins University Press, 2011.

Chan, Lawrence C.N., Hon M. Cheung, Terence C.W. Poon, Terence P.Y. Ma, Hugh S. Lam, Pak C. Ng. "End-of-Life Decision-Making for Newborns: A 12-year Experience in Hong Kong." *Archives of Disease in Childhood: Fetal and Neonatal Edition* 101, no. 1 (2016): F37–F42.

Cherry, Mark J. "Ignoring the Data and Endangering Children: Why the Mature Minor Standard for Medical Decision Making Must Be Abandoned." *Journal of Medicine and Philosophy* 38, no. 3 (2013): 315–331.

Cherry, Mark J. "The Consumerist Moral Babel of the Post-Modern Family." Christian *Bioethics* 21, no. 2 (2015): 144–165.

Chochinov, Harvey Max, Keith G. Wilson, Murray Enns, Neil Mowchun, Sheila Lander, Martin Levitt, and Jennifer J. Clinch. "Desire for Death in the Terminally Ill." *American Journal of Psychiatry* 152 (1995): 1185–1191.

Cochran, Donald, Sarosh Saleem, Sumaira Khowaja-Punjwani, John D. Lantos. "Cross-Cultural Differences in Communication about a Dying Child." *Pediatrics* 140, no. 5 (2017): e20170690.

Contro, Nancy A., Judith Larson, Sarah Scofield, Barbara Sourkes, and Harvey J. Cohen. "Hospital Staff and Family Perspectives Regarding Quality of Pediatric Palliative Care." *Pediatrics* 114, no. 5 (2004): 1248–1252.

Contro, Nancy A., Judith Larson, Sarah Scofield, Barbara Sourkes, and Harvey J. Cohen. "Family Perspectives on the Quality of Pediatric Palliative Care." *Archives of Pediatrics & Adolescent Medicine* 156, no. 1 (2002): 14–19.

Cook, Michael. "Dutch pediatricians seek child euthanasia," *National Right to Life News*, (2016): 42.

Cook, Sarah Sheets, ed. *Children and Dying: An Exploration and a Selective Bibliography*. New York: Health Sciences Publishing Corporation, 1973.

Cooper, John M. "Stoic Autonomy." *Social Philosophy and Policy* 20, no. 2 (2003): 1–29.

Coyne, Imelda and Lisa Kirwan. "Ascertaining Children's Wishes and Feelings about Hospital Life." *Journal of Child Health Care* 16, no. 3 (2012): 293–304.

Coyne, Imelda. "Consultation With Children in Hospital: Children, Parents' and Nurses' Perspectives." *Journal of Clinical Nursing* 15, no. 1 (2006) 61–71.

Coyne, Imelda. "Response." *Journal of Clinical Nursing* 15, no. 6 (2006), 794.

Dan, Bernard, Christine Fonteyne, Stéphan Clément de Cléty. "Self-requested euthanasia for children in Belgium." *The Lancet* 383, no. 9918 (2014): 671–672.

Davies, Betty, John B. Collins, Rose Steele, Karen Cook, Amy Brenner, and Stephany Smith. "Children's Perspectives of a Pediatric Hospice Program." *Journal of Palliative Care* 21, no. 4 (2005): 252–261.

Davies, Dawn. "Medical Assistance in Dying: A Paediatric Perspective." *Paediatrics & Child Health* (2018): 125–130.

De Vos, Mirjam A., Agnes van der Heide, Heleen Maurice-Stam, Oebele F. Brouwer, Frans B. Plötz, Antoinette Y. N. Schouten-van Meeteren, Dick L. Willems, Hugo S. A. Heymans, and Albert P. Bos. "The Process of End-of-Life Decision-Making in Pediatrics: A National Survey in the Netherlands." *Pediatrics* 127, no. 4 (2011): e1004–e1012.

DeMichelis, Carey, Randi Zlotnik Shaul, and Adam Rapoport. "Medical Assistance in Dying at a Paediatric Hospital." *Journal of Medical Ethics* 45 (2019): 60–67.

Derrington, Susan. "Are We Doing Right by Dying Children?" *The Journal of Paediatrics* 166 (2015): 524–525.

Dillen, Annemie, and Didier Pollefeyt, eds. *Children's Voices: Children's Perspectives in Ethics, Theology and Religious Education*. Leuven: Uitgeverij Peeters, 2010.

Doran, Robert M. *Theology and the Dialectics of History*. Toronto: University of Toronto Press, 1990.

Drake, Ross, Judy Frost, and John J. Collins. "The Symptoms of Dying Children." *Journal of Pain and Symptom Management* 26 (2003): 594–603.

Duffin, Jaclyn. *History of Medicine: A Scandalously Short Introduction*. 2nd ed. Toronto: University of Toronto Press, 2010.

Dussel, Veronica, Ulrika Kreicbergs, Joanne M. Hilden, Jan Watterson, Caron Moore, Brian G. Turner, Jane C. Weeks, and Joanne Wolfe. "Looking Beyond Where Children Die: Determinants and Effects of Planning a Child's Location of Death." *Journal of Pain and Symptom Management* 37, no. 1 (2009): 33–43.

Elliot, Carl. *Better Than Well: American Medicine Meets the American Dream*. New York: W. W. Norton: 2004.

Ely, Elizabeth A. "The Experience of Pain for School-Age Children: Blood, Band-Aids, and Feelings." *Children's Health Care* 21 (1992): 168–176.

Engelhardt, Tristram H. "Beyond the Best Interests of Children: Four Views of the Family and of Foundational Disagreements Regarding Pediatric Decision Making." *Journal of Medicine and Philosophy* 35 (2010): 499–517.

Ernst, Michelle M., Carrie Piazza-Waggoner, and Heather Ciesielski. "The Role of Pediatric Psychologists in Facilitating Medical Decision Making in the Care of Critically Ill Young Children." *Clinical Practice in Pediatric Psychology* 3, no. 2 (2015): 120–130.

Evans, John H. *Playing God?: Human Genetic Engineering and the Rationalization of Public Bioethical Discourse*. Chicago: University of Chicago Press, 2002.

Feudtner, Chris, Jeff Haney, and Martha A. Dimmers. "Spiritual Care Needs of Hospitalized Children and Their Families: A National Survey of Pastoral Care Providers' Perceptions." *Pediatrics* 111, no. 1 (2003): e67–72.

Foot, Philippa. *Natural Goodness*. Oxford: Oxford University Press, 2001.

Francis, James M. M. *Adults as Children: Images of Childhood in the Ancient World and the New Testament*. New York: Peter Lang, 2006.

Furingsten, Lovisa, Reet Sjögren, and Maria Forsner. "Ethical Challenges When Caring for Dying Children." *Nursing Ethics* 22, no. 2 (2015): 176–187.

Gandolfo, Elizabeth O'Donnell. *The Power and Vulnerability of Love: A Theological Anthropology*. Minneapolis: Fortress Press, 2015.

Garroway, Kristine Henriksen. *Growing up in Ancient Israel: Children in Material Culture and Biblical Texts*. Atlanta: SBL Press, 2018.

Gendlin, Eugene. *Experiencing and the Creation of Meaning: A Philosophical and Psychological Approach to the Subjective.* Evanston: Northwestern University Press, 1997.

Gill, C. "The False Autonomy of Forced Choice: Rationalizing Suicide for Persons with Disabilities." *Contemporary Perspectives on Rational Suicide,* edited by J. L. Werth, 171–180. New York: Taylor & Francis, 1999.

Golden, Mark. *Children and Childhood in Classical Athens.* 2nd ed. Baltimore: Johns Hopkins University Press, 2015.

Goldhagen, Jeffrey, Paul Mercer, Elspeth Webb, Rita Nathawad, Sherry Shenoda, and Gerison Lansdown. "Toward a Child Rights Theory in Pediatric Bioethics." *Perspectives in Biology and Medicine* 58, no. 3 (2015): 306–319.

Goldhill, Simon. "A Mother's Joy at Her Child's Death: Conversion, Cognitive Dissonance, and Grief." *Victorian Studies* 59, no. 4 (2017): 636–657.

Green, Melody. "Death and Nonsense in the Poetry of George MacDonald's *At the Back of the North Wind* and Lewis Carroll's *Alice* Books." *North Wind: A Journal of George MacDonald Studies* 30, no. 4 (2011): 38–49.

Guyer, Paul. "Kant on the Theory and Practice of Autonomy." *Social Philosophy and Policy* 20, no. 2 (2003): 70–98.

Guylay, Jo-Eileen. *The Dying Child.* Toronto: McGraw-Hill, 1978.

Harmic, Ann B., John D. Arras, and Margaret E. Mohrmann. "Must We Be Courageous?" *Hastings Center Report* 45, no. 3 (2015): 33–40.

Hart, Roger A. *Children's Participation: From Tokenism to Citizenship.* Innocenti Essays 4. Florence, Italy: International Child Development Centre, 1992.

Hauerwas, Stanley. *God, Medicine, and Suffering.* Grand Rapids, MI: Eerdmans, 1990.

———. *The Hauerwas Reader.* Edited by John Berkman and Michael Cartwright. Durham: Duke University Press, 2001.

———. "Situation Ethics, Moral Notions, and Moral Theology." In *Vision and Virtue: Essays in Christian Ethical Reflection.* Notre Dame: University of Notre Dame Press, 1974.

———. *Suffering Presence: Theological Reflections on Medicine, the Mentally Handicapped, and the Church.* Notre Dame, IN: University of Notre Dame Press, 1986.

Heaps, Jonathan. "Insight is a Body-feeling: Experiencing our Understanding." *The Heythrop Journal* 57, no. 3 (2015): 1–12.

Hedie, Agnes van der, Luc Deliens, Karin Faisst, Tore Nilstun, Michael Norup, Eugenio Paci, Gerrit van der Wal, Paul J van der Maas. "End-of-Life Decision-Making in Six European Countries: Descriptive Study." *The Lancet* 361, no. 9381 (2003): 35–350.

Hein, Irma M., Pieter W. Troost, Martine C. de Vries, Catherijne A.J. Knibbe, Johannes B. van Goudoever, and Ramón J.L. Lindauer. "Why Do Children Decide Not to Participate in Clinical Research: A Quantitative and Qualitative Study?" *Pediatric Research* 78, no. 1 (2015): 103–108.

Heinze, Katherine E., and Marie T. Nolan. "Parental Decision Making for Children With Cancer at the End of Life: A Meta-Ethnography." *Journal of Pediatric Oncology Nursing* 29, no. 6 (November 2012): 337–345.

Herdt, Jennifer A. *Putting on Virtue: The Legacy of the Splendid Vices*. Chicago: University of Chicago Press, 2008.

Herzog, Kristin. *Children and Our Global Future: Theological and Social Challenges*. Cleveland: Pilgrim Press, 2005.

Hettema, Theo L. "Autonomy and Its Vulnerability: Ricoeur's View on Justice as a Contribution to Care Ethics." *Medicine, Health Care and Philosophy* 17, no. 4 (2014): 493–498.

Hill, B. Jessie. "Whose body? Whose soul? Medical Decision-Making on Behalf of Children and the Free Exercise Clause before and after *Employment Division v. Smith*." *Cardozo Law Review* 32, no. 5 (2011): 1857–1878.

Hill, Douglas L., Victoria A. Miller, Kari R. Hexem, Karen W. Carroll, Jennifer A. Faerber, Tammy Kang, and Chris Feudtner. "Problems and Hopes Perceived by Mothers, Fathers and Physicians of Children Receiving Palliative Care." *Health Expectations* 18, no. 5 (2015): 1052–1065.

Hinds, Pamela S., Lisa Schum, Justin N. Baker, and Joanne Wolfe. "Key Factors Affecting Dying Children and Their Families." *Journal of Palliative Medicine* 8, no. 1 (2005): S70–S78.

Hinson, Ashley P., and Philip M. Rosoff. "Where Children Die: Obstacles to Qualify End-of-Life Care." *Clinical Pediatrics* 55, no. 2 (2015): 101–106.

Horn, Cornelia B. and John W. Martens. *"Let the Little Children Come to Me": Childhood and Children in Early Christianity*. Washington, DC: The Catholic University of America Press, 2009.

Hoffmaster, Barry. "The Rationality and Morality of Dying Children." *The Hastings Center Report* 41, no. 6 (2011): 30–42.

Hui, Edwin. "Parental Refusal of Life-Saving Treatments for Adolescents: Chinese Familism in Medical Decision-Making Revisited." *Bioethics* 22 (2008): 286–295.

Humphry, Derek. *Dying with Dignity: Understanding Euthanasia.* New York: Birch Lane Press, 1992.

Hynson J.L., R. Aroni, C. Bauld, and S.M. Sawyer. "Research with Bereaved Parents: A Question of How Not Why." *Palliative Medicine* 20, no. 8 (2006): 805–811.

Jacobs, Jonathan. "Some Tensions between Autonomy and Self-Governance." *Social Philosophy and Policy* 20, no. 2 (2003): 221–244.

Jalmsell, Li, Taru Kontino, Maria Stein, Jan-Inge Henter, and Ulrika Kreicbergs. "On the Child's Own Initiative: Parents Communicate with Their Dying Child About Death." *Death Studies* 39, no. 2 (2015): 111–117.

Jankovic, Momcilo, John J. Spinetta, Giuseppe Masera, Ronald D. Barr, Giulio J. D'Angio, Claudia Epelman, Audrey Evans, Helen Vasilatou Kosmidis, and Tim Eden. "Communicating with the Dying Child: An Invitation to Listening—A Report of the SIOP Working Committee on Psychosocial Issues in Pediatric Oncology." *Pediatric Blood and Cancer* 50 (2008): 1087–1088.

Jensen, Claus Sixtus, Karen Jackson, Raymond Kolbæk, and Stinne Glasdam. "Children's Experiences of Acute Hospitalisation to a Paediatric Emergency and Assessment Unit—A Qualitative Study." *Journal of Child Health Care* 16, no. 3 (2012): 263–273.

Jensen, David H. *Graced Vulnerability: A Theology of Childhood.* Cleveland: Pilgrim Press, 2005.

Jeremic, Vida, Karine Sénécal, Pascal Borry, Davit Chokoshvili, and Danya F. Vears. "Participation of Children in Medical Decision-Making: Challenges and Potential Solutions." *Bioethical Inquiry* 13, no. 4 (2016): 525–534.

Jerrett, Mary D. "Children and Their Pain Experience." *Children's Health Care* 14, no. 2 (1985): 83–89.

Jesson, Stuart. "Simone Weil: Suffering, Attention and Compassionate Thought." *Studies in Christian Ethics* 27, no. 2 (2014): 185–201.

Jolley, Jeremy. "Commentary on Coyne I (2006) Consultation with Children in Hospital: Children, Parents' and Nurses' Perspectives, Journal of Clinical Nursing 15 61–71." *Journal of Clinical Nursing* 15, no. 6 (2006): 791–793.

Kane, Javier R., Melody Brown Hellsten, Rev. April Coldsmith. "Human Suffering: The Need for Relationship-Based Research in Pediatric End-of-Life Care." *Journal of Pediatric Oncology Nursing* 21, no. 3 (2004): 180–185.

Kant, Immanuel. *Anthropology from a Pragmatic Point of View*. Translated and Edited by Robert B. Louden. Cambridge: Cambridge University Press, 2006.

———. *Groundwork of the Metaphysics of Morals*. Translated and Edited by Mary Gregor and Jens Timmerman. Cambridge: Cambridge University Press, 2012.

Kaveny, Cathleen. *Law's Virtues: Fostering Autonomy and Solidarity in American Society*. Washington, DC: Georgetown University Press, 2012.

Keele, Linda, Heather T. Keenan, Joan Sheetz, and Susan L. Bratton. "Differences in Characteristics of Dying Children Who Receive and Do Not Receive Palliative Care." *Pediatrics* 132, no. 1 (2013): 72–78.

Klein, Scott M. "Moral Distress in Pediatric Palliative Care: A Case Study." *Journal of Pain and Symptom Management* 38, no. 1 (2009): 157–160.

Kopelman, Loretta M., and John C. Moskop. *Children and Health Care: Moral and Social Issues*. Boston: Kluwer Academic Publishers, 1989.

Kovesi, Julius. *Moral Notions*. London: Rutledge, 1971.

Kramer, Kenneth. "You Cannot Die Alone: Dr. Elisabeth Kübler-Ross (July 8, 1926–August 24, 2004)." *OMEGA—Journal of Death and Dying* 50, no. 2 (2005): 83–101.

Kreicbergs, Ulrika, Lilian Pohlkamp, and Josefin Sveen. "No Impact of Previous Evidence Advocating Openness to Talk to Children about Their Imminent Death." *Acta Paediatrica* 110, no. 5 (2021): 1671–1672.

Kreicbergs, Ulrika, Unnur Valdimarsdóttir, Erik Onelöv, Jan-Inge Henter, and Gunnar Steineck. "Talking about Death with Children Who Have Severe Malignant Disease." *The New England Journal of Medicine* 351, no. 12 (2004): 1175–1186.

Kreicbergs, Ulrika. "Why and Where Do Children Die?" *Acta Pædiatrica* 107, no. 10 (2018): 1671–1672.

Kübler-Ross, Elisabeth. *On Children and Death: How Children and Their Parents Can and Do Cope with Death*. New York: Touchstone Books. 1997.

Kudryavtsev, Vladimir. "The Imagination of the Preschool Child: The Experience of Logical-Psychological Analysis." *Journal of Russian & East European Psychology* 54, nos. 4–5 (2017): 393–401.

Langworthy, Rebecca. "Crossing that Great Frontier: Transformative Reading in Phantastes and C.S. Lewis' Perelandra." *North Wind: A Journal of George MacDonald Studies* 36, no. 5 (2017): 87–95.

Lantos, John, ed. *The Ethics of Shared Decision Making.* Oxford: Oxford University Press, 2021.

Lancy, David F. *The Anthropology of Childhood: Cherubs, Chattel, Changelings* 2nd ed. Cambridge: Cambridge University Press, 2014.

Laqueur, Thomas W. *The Work of the Dead: A Cultural History of Mortal Remains.* Princeton: Princeton University Press, 2015.

Lawrence, Penny. "Hearing and Acting with the Voices of Children in Early Childhood." *Journal of the British Academy* 8, no. 4 (2022): 77–90.

Leenen, Catelijne. "Children's Rights and the Dutch Termination of Life on Request and Assisted Suicide (Review Procedures) Act." In *Developmental and Autonomy Rights in Children: Empowering Children, Caregivers and Communities.* Edited by Jan C. M. Willems, 141–164. New York: Intersentia, 2002.

Lehrer, Keith. "Reason and Autonomy." *Social Philosophy and Policy* 20, no. 2 (2003): 177–98.

Lewis, C. S. "On Three Ways of Writing for Children." In *Of Other Worlds: Essays and Stories.* Edited by Walter Hooper. New York: Harcourt, Brace, & World, 1967.

Lin, Jody L., Catherine L. Clark, Bonnie Halpern-Felsher, Paul N. Bennett, Shiri Assis-Hassid, Ofra Amir, Yadira Castaneda Nunez, Nancy Miles Cleary, Sebastian Gehrmann, Barbara J. Grosz and Lee M. Sanders. "Parent Perspectives in Shared Decision-Making for Children With Medical Complexity." *Academic Pediatrics* 20, no. 8 (2020): 1101–1108.

Lipstein, Ellen A., William B. Brinkman, Alexander G. Fiks, Kristin S. Hendrix, Jennifer Kryworuchko, Victoria A. Miller, Lisa A. Prosser, Wendy J. Ungar and David Fox. "An Emerging Field of Research: Challenges in Pediatric Decision Making." *Medical Decision Making* 35, no. 3 (2015): 403–408.

van Loenhout, Rhiannon B., Ivana M. M. van der Geest, Astrid M. Vrakking, Agnes van der Heide, Rob Pieters, Marry M. van den Heuvel-Eibrink. "End-of-Life Decisions in Pediatric Cancer Patients." *Journal of Palliative Medicine* 18, no. 8 (2015): 697–702.

Lonergan, Bernard. *Insight.* Vol. 3, *The Collected Works of Bernard Lonergan.* Toronto: University of Toronto Press, 1988.

———. *Method in Theology.* Toronto: University of Toronto Press, 1990.

———. *Topics in Education.* Vol. 10, *The Collected Works of Bernard Lonergan.* Toronto: University of Toronto Press, 2000.

Lövgren, Malin, Christina Melin-Johansson, Camilla Udo, and Josefin Sveen. "Telling the Truth to Dying Children—End-of-Life Communication with Families." *Acta Pædiatrica* 108, no. 11 (2019): 2111–2112.

von Lützau, Pia, Michael Otto, Tanja Hechler, Sabine Metzing, Joanne Wolfe, and Boris Zernikow. "Children Dying from Cancer: Parents' Perspective on Symptoms, Quality of Life, Characteristics of Death, and End-of-Life Decisions." *Journal of Palliative Care* 28, no. 4 (2012): 274–281.

Lysaught, Theresa M., Joseph Kotva, Stephen E. Lammers and AllenVerhey, eds. *On Moral Medicine: Theological Perspectives in Medical Ethics.* Grand Rapids: Eerdmans, 1998.

MacDonald, George. *At the Back of the North Wind.* London: Alfred A. Knopf, 2001.

———. *The Complete Fairy Tales.* Edited by U. C. Knoepflmacher. New York: Penguin Books, 1999.

———. "The Imagination: Its Function and Its Culture." In *A Dish of Orts. Chiefly Papers on the Imagination, and on Shakespeare,* 1–42. London: Sampson Low Maston & Company, 1893.

———. *Phantastes: A Faerie Romance.* New York: Dover Publications Inc., 2005.

———. *The Princess and the Goblin.* London: Puffin Classics, 2010.

MacDonald, Greville, ed. *George MacDonald and His Wife.* London: Johannesen Publishing, 1998.

MacIntyre, Alasdair. *After Virtue.* 3rd ed. Notre Dame, IN: Notre Dame University Press, 2007.

Mackenzie, Catriona and Natalie Stoljar, ed. *Relational Autonomy: Feminist Perspectives on Autonomy, Agency, and the Social Self.* New York: Oxford University Press, 2000.

Margherita, G., M. L. Martino, F. Recano and F. Camera. "Invented Fairy Tales in Groups with Onco-Haematological Children." *Child: Care, Health and Development* 40 (2014): 426–427.

Massmann, Alexander. "Genetic Enhancements and Relational Autonomy: Christian Ethics and the Child's Autonomy in Vulnerability." *Studies in Christian Ethics* 32, no. 1 (2018): 88–104.

Matthews, Gareth B. *Conversations with Children.* Cambridge: Harvard University Press, 1984.

———, and Susan M. Turner, eds. *The Philosopher's Child: Critical Perspectives in the Western Tradition*. Rochester: University of Rochester Press, 1998.

———. *Philosophy and the Young Child*. Cambridge: Harvard University Press, 1980.

———. *The Philosophy of Childhood*. Cambridge: Harvard University Press, 1994.

Mattson, Craig E. and Virginia LaGrand. "Eros at the World's End: Apocalyptic Attention in the Love Stories of Graham Greene and P. D. James," *Renascence* 64 no. 3 (2012): 275–294.

Maurer, Scott H., Pamela S. Hinds, Sheri L. Spunt, Wayne L. Furman, Javier R. Kane, and Justin N. Baker. "Decision Making by Parents of Children with Incurable Cancer Who Opt for Enrollment on a Phase I Trial Compared with Choosing a Do Not Resuscitate/Terminal Care Option." *Journal of Clinical Oncology* 28, no. 20 (2010): 3292–3298.

McCabe, Mary Ann. "Involving Children and Adolescents in Medical Decision Making: Developmental and Clinical Considerations." *Journal of Paediatric Psychology* 21, no. 4 (1996): 505–516.

McCallum, Dawn E., Paul Byrne, and Eduardo Bruera. "How Children Die in Hospital." *Journal of Pain and Symptom Management* 20, no. 6 (2000): 417–423.

McEvoy, James Gerard. "Theology of Childhood: An Essential Element of Christian Anthropology." *Irish Theological Quarterly* 84, no. 2 (2019): 117–136.

McGavock, Karen L. "Agents of Reform?: Children's Literature and Philosophy." *Philosophia* 35, no. B (2007): 129–143.

McGillis, Roderick. "'A Fairytale is Just a Fairytale': George MacDonald and the Queering of Fairy." *Marvels & Tales* 17 (2003): 86–99.

Meilaender, Gilbert. *Bioethics: A Primer for Christians*. Grand Rapids: Eerdmans, 2005.

Melin-Johanosson, Christina, Inge Axelsson, Marie Jonsson Grundberg, and Frida Hallqvist. "When a Child Dies: Parents' Experiences of Palliative Care—An Integrative Literature Review." *Journal of Pediatric Nursing* 29, no. 6 (2014): 660–669.

Mercer, Joyce Ann. *Welcoming Children: A Practical Theology of Childhood*. St. Louis: Chalice Press, 2005.

Miller, Geoffrey, ed. *Pediatric Bioethics*. Cambridge: Cambridge University Press, 2010.

Miller, Mark T. *The Quest for God and the Good Life: Lonergan's Theological Anthropology.* Washington, DC: Catholic University of America Press, 2013.

Miller, Richard B. *Children, Ethics, and Modern Medicine.* Indianapolis: Indiana University Press, 2003.

Miller-McLemore, Bonnie J. *Let the Children Come: Reimagining Childhood from a Christian Perspective.* San Francisco: Jossey-Bass, 2003.

Mitchell, J. Allan. *Becoming Human: The Matter of the Medieval Child.* Minneapolis: University of Minnesota Press, 2014.

Mohrmann, Margaret. *Attending Children: A Doctor's Education.* Washington, DC: Georgetown University Press, 2006.

———, and Lois Shepherd. "Ready to Listen: Why Welcome Matters." *Journal of Pain and Symptom Management* 43, no. 3 (2012): 646–650.

———. "Whose Interests Are They, Anyway?" *Journal of Religious Ethics* 34, no. 1 (2006): 141–150.

Moltmann, Jurgen. "Child and Childhood as Metaphors of Hope." *Theology Today* 56, no. 4 (2000): 592–603.

Montgomery, Heather. *An Introduction to Childhood: Anthropological Perspectives on Children's Lives.* Chichester: Wiley-Blackwell, 2009.

Mukhida, Karim. "Loving Your Child to Death: Considerations of the Care of Chronically Ill Children and Euthanasia in Emil Sher's *Mourning Dove.*" *Pediatric Child Health* 12, no. 10 (2007): 859–865.

Newey, Edmund. *Children of God: The Child as Source of Theological Anthropology.* Burlington: Ashgate, 2012.

Newton, Hannah. "The Dying Child in Seventeenth-Century England." *Pediatrics* 136, no. 2 (2015): 218–220.

Niethammer, Dietrich. *Speaking Honestly with Sick And Dying Children and Adolescents: Unlocking the Silence.* Translated by Victoria W. Hill. Baltimore: Johns Hopkins University Press, 2012.

Nilsson, Stefan, Berit Björkman, Anna-Lena Almqvist, Lena Almqvist, Polly Björk-Willén, Dana Donohue, Karin Enskär, Mats Granlund, Karina Huus, & Sara Hvit. "Children's Voices – Differentiating a Child Perspective from a Child's Perspective." *Developmental Neurorehabilitation* 18, no. 3 (2015): 162–168.

van Nistelrooij, Inge, Petruschka Schaafsma, and Joan C. Tronto. "Ricoeur and the Ethics of Care." *Medicine, Health Care and Philosophy* 17, no. 4 (2014): 485–491.

Nova, Cristina, Elena Vegni, Egidio Aldo Moja. "The Physician–Patient–Parent Communication: A Qualitative Perspective on the Child's Contribution." *Patient Education and Counseling* 58, no. 3 (2005): 327–333.

Nussbaum, Abraham M. "Discipleship, Nonresistance, and the Communal Care of People With Mental Illness in Late 20th-Century America." *The Journal of Nervous and Mental Disease* 200, no. 12 (2012): 1088–1094.

O'Donovan, Oliver. *Finding and Seeing*. Vol 2, *Ethics as Theology*. Grand Rapids: Eerdmans, 2014.

———. *Self, World, and Time*. Vol 1, *Ethics as Theology*. Grand Rapids: Eerdmans, 2013.

Orme, Nicholas. *Medieval Children*. New Haven: Yale University Press, 2001.

Oshana, Marina. "How Much Should We Value Autonomy?" *Social Philosophy and Policy* 20, no. 2 (2003): 99–126.

Ott, Kate. "Taking Children's Moral Lives Seriously: Creativity as Ethical Response Offline and Online." *Religions* 10, no. 525 (2019): 1–12.

Parker, Julie Faith. *Valuable and Vulnerable: Children in the Hebrew Bible, Especially the Elisha Cycle*. Providence: Brown University, 2013.

Partridge, Brian C. "The Decisional Capacity of the Adolescent: An Introduction to a Critical Reconsideration of the Doctrine of the Mature Minor." *Journal of Medicine and Philosophy* 38, no. 3 (2013): 249–255.

Pasulka, Diana. "A Somber Pedagogy—A History of the Child Death Bed Scene in Early American Children's Religious Literature, 1674–1840." *The Journal of the History of Childhood and Youth* 2 (2009): 171–197.

Paul, Ellen Frankel, Fred D. Miller Jr., and Jeffrey Paul eds. *Autonomy*. Cambridge: Cambridge University Press, 2010.

Pazdziora, Patrick J. "'The Path of Pain' George MacDonald's Portrayal of Death in The Diary of an Old Soul." *North Wind: A Journal of George MacDonald Studies* 36, no. 6 (2017): 96–117.

Pelizzo, Gloria, Valeria Calcaterra, Selene Ostuni, Marco Ferraresi, and Maria Rita Parsi. "Child's Suffering: Proposals to Support and Manage the Illness." *Journal of Medicine and the Person* 12, no. 2 (2014): 84–90.

Pelto-Piri, Veikko, Karin Engström, and Ingemar Engström. "Paternalism, Autonomy and Reciprocity: Ethical Perspectives in Encounters with Patients in Psychiatric In-patient Care." *BMC Medical Ethics* 14, no. 49 (2013): 1–8.

Pemberton, Marilyn. "The Ultimate Rite of Passage: Death and Beyond in 'The Golden Key' and *At the Back of the North Wind*." *North Wind: A Journal of George MacDonald Studies* 27, no. 3 (2008): 35–50.

Peterson, Jane. W. and Yvonne M. Sterling. "Children's Perceptions of Asthma: African American Children Use Metaphors to Make Sense of Asthma." *Journal of Paediatric Health Care* 23, no. 2 (2009): 93–100.

Pfund, Rita and Susan Fowler-Kerry, eds., *Perspectives on Palliative Care for Children and Young People: A Global Discourse*. New York: Radcliffe Publishing, 2010.

Piaget, Jean. *The Child's Conception of the World*. Translated by Joan and Andrew Tomlinson. New York: Rowman & Littlefied, 2007.

———. *The Origins of Intelligence in Children*. Translated by Margaret Cook. New York: Norton, 1963.

Pickup, Mark. "The Murder of Tracy Latimer." *Human Life Review* 27, no. 2 (2001): 1–9.

Pinches, Charles. "Principle Monism and Action Descriptions: Situationism and its Critics Revisited," *Modern Theology* 7 (1991): 249–268.

———. *Theology and Action: After Theory in Christian Ethics*. Grand Rapids: Eerdmans, 2002.

Pinckaers, Servais. *The Pinckaers Reader: Renewing Thomistic Moral Theology*. Edited by John Berkman and Craig Steven Titus. Washington, DC: The Catholic University of America Press, 2005.

Plebanek, Daniel J., and Vladimir M. Sloutsky. "Costs of Selective Attention: When Children Notice What Adults Miss." *Psychological Science* 28, no. 6 (2017): 723–732.

Pridmore, John. "George Macdonald's Estimate of Childhood." *International Journal of Children's Spirituality* 12, no. 1 (2007): 61–74.

Pritchard, Michele, Elizabeth A. Burghen, Jami S. Gattuso, Nancy K. West, Poorna Gajjar, Deo Kumar Srivastava, Sheri L. Spunt et al. "Factors That Distinguish Symptoms of Most Concern to Parents from Other Symptoms of Dying Children." *Journal of Pain and Symptom Management* 39, no. 4 (2010): 627–636.

Prugh, Dane G., Elizabeth M. Staub, Harriet H. Sands, Ruth M. Kirschbaum, and Ellenora A. Lenihan. "A Study of the Emotional Reactions of Children and Families to Hospitalization and Illness." *American Journal of Orthopsychiatry* 23, no. 1 (1953): 70–106.

Punt, Jeremy. "Not Child's Play: Paul and Children." Neotestamentica 51, no. 2 (2017): 235–259.

Pyper, Hugh. "Children." In *The Oxford Companion to Christian Thought*, edited by Adrian Hastings, 100. Oxford: Oxford University Press, 2000.

Rahner, Karl. "Ideas for a Theology of Childhood." In *Theological Investigations.* Vol. 8, *Further Theology of the Spiritual Life 2.* Translated by David Bourke, 33–50. New York: Herder and Herder, 1971.

Ramaswamy, Sheila, and Shekhar Seshadri. "Our Failure to Protect Sexually Abused Children: Where Is Our 'Willing Suspension of Disbelief'?" *Indian Journal of Psychiatry* 59, no. 2 (2017): 233–235.

Ramnarayan, Padmanabhan, Finella Craig, Andy Petros, Christine Pierce. "Characteristics of Deaths Occurring in Hospitalised Children: Changing Trends." *Journal of Medical Ethics* 33, no. B (2007): 255–260.

Ramos, Rui, and Ana Margarida Ramos. "Children's Literature and the Promotion of Environmental Ethics in Portugal." *Portugese Studies* 31, no. 1 (2015): 94–106.

Recchia, Susan L., Minsun Shin, and Carolina Snaider. "Where is the Love? Developing Loving Relationships as an Essential Component of Professional Infant Care." *International Journal of Early Years Education* 26, no. 2 (2018): 142–158.

Reinders, Hans S. *Receiving the Gift of Friendship: Profound Disability, Theological Anthropology, and Ethics.* Grand Rapids: Eerdmans, 2008.

Renjilian, C.B., James W. Womer, Karen W. Carroll, Tammy I. Kang, and Chris Feudtner. "Parental Explicit Heuristics in Decision-Making for Children With Life-Threatening Illnesses." *Pediatrics* 131, no. 2 (2013): 566–572.

Reynolds, Thomas. *Vulnerable Communion: A Theology of Disability and Hospitality.* Grand Rapids: Brazos Press, 2008.

Richards, Anne and Peter Privett, eds. *Through the Eyes of a Child: New Insights in Theology from a Child's Perspective.* London: Church House Publishing, 2009.

Ricoeur, Paul. *Oneself as Another.* Translated by Kathleen Blamey. Chicago: University of Chicago Press, 1992.

Riem, Madelon M.E., van IJzendoorn, M. H., De Carli, P., Vingerhoets, A. J. J. M., and Bakermans-Kranenburg, M. J. "Behavioural and Neural Responses to Infant and Adult Tears: The Impact of Maternal Love Withdrawal." *Emotion* 17, no. 6 (2017): 1021–1029.

van der Riet, Pamela, Chaweewan Jitsacorn, Piyatida Junlapeeya, and Peter Thursby. "Student Nurses Experience of a 'Fairy Garden' Healing Haven Garden for Sick Children." *Nurse Education Today* 59 (2017): 88–93.

Rini, Annie, and Lillia Loriz. "Anticipatory Mourning in Parents With a Child Who Dies Whilst Hospitalized." *Journal of Pediatric Nursing* 22, no. 4 (2007): 272–282.

Rokash, Ami and Maneli Parvini. "Experience of Adults and Children in Hospitals." *Early Child Development and Care* 181 no. 5 (2011): 707–715.

Römer, Thomas C. "Why Would the Deuteronomists Tell About the Sacrifice of Jephthah's Daughter?" *Journal for the Study of the Old Testament* 77 (1998): 27–38.

Rousseau, Jean-Jacques. *Emile or On Education.* Translated by Allan Bloom. New York: Basic Books, 1979.

Rubio, Julie Hanlon. "The Dual Vocation of Christian Parents." *Theological Studies* 63, no. 4 (2002): 786–812.

Ruhe, Katharina, M., Eva De Clercq, Tenzin Wangmo, and Bernice S. Elger. "Relational Capacity: Broadening the Notion of Decision-Making Capacity in Paediatric Healthcare." *Bioethical Inquiry* 16, no. 13 (2016): 515–524.

Runeson, I., E. Mårtensson, and K. Enskär. "Children's Knowledge and Degree of Participating in Decision Making When Undergoing a Clinical Diagnostic Procedure." *Pediatric Nursing* 33, no. 6 (2007): 505–511.

Rust, Val D. "The Policy Formation Process and Educational Reform in Norway." *Comparative Education* 26, no. 1 (1990): 13–25.

Ryan, E. E. "Aristotle's Rhetoric and Ethics and the Ethos of Society." *Greek Roman and Byzantine Studies* 13 (1972): 291–308.

Ryan, Maura A. "The Politics of Risk: A Human Rights Paradigm for Children's Environmental Health Research." *Environmental Health Perspectives* 114, no. 10 (2006): 1613–1616.

Salter, Erica K. "Reimagining Childhood: Responding to the Challenge Presented by Severe Developmental Disability." *Hospital Ethics Committee Forum* 29, (2017): 241–256.

Salvey, Courtney. "Riddled with Evil: Fantasy as Theodicy in George MacDonald's Phantastes and Lilith." *North Wind: A Journal of George MacDonald Studies* 27, no. 2 (2008): 16–34.

Sanchez Varela, Ana M., Liza-Marie Johnson, Javier R. Kane, Kimberly A. Kasow, Yuri Quintana, April Coan, Ying Yuan, Raymond Barfield, Christopher Church, Micah Hester, and Justin N. Baker. "Ethical Decision Making about End-of-Life Care Issues by Pediatric Oncologists in Economically Diverse Settings." *Journal of Pediatric Hematology/Oncology* 37, no. 4 (2015): 257–263.

Sautereau, Cyndie. "Subjectivité et vulnérabilité chez Ricœur et Levinas." *Études Ricœuriennes* 4, no. 2 (2013): 8–24.

Scheper-Hughes, Nancy, and Carolyn Fishel Sargent. *Small Wars: The Cultural Politics of Childhood.* Berkeley: University of California Press, 1998.

Shier-Jones, Angela, ed. *Children of God: Towards a Theology of Children.* Peterborough: Epworth, 2007.

Schneewind, J. B. *The Invention of Autonomy.* Cambridge: Cambridge University Press, 1998.

Sedgwick, Sally. *Kant's Groundwork of the Metaphysics of Morals: An Introduction.* Cambridge: Cambridge University Press, 2008.

Shakespeare, Tom. *Disability Rights and Wrongs.* London: Routledge, 2006.

Sheldon, Mark. "Medical Decision-Making for Children and the Question of Legitimate Authority." *Theoretical Medicine and Bioethics* 25, no. 4 (2004): 225–228.

Shuman, Joel and Brian Volck. *Reclaiming the Body: Christians and the Faithful Use of Modern Medicine.* Grand Rapids: Brazos Press, 2006.

Slaninka, M., P. Krajmer, and A. Kolenova. "Main Topics Related to the Disease, Death, and Dying in Communication between Parents and Their Adolescent Children with Incurable Cancer." *Bratislava Medical Journal* 122, no. 8 (2021): 572–576.

Smith, Izetta. "Preschool Children 'Play' out Their Grief." *Death Studies* 15, no. 2 (1991): 169–176.

Soyinka, Wole. "Ethics, Bio-ethics and Environment in Healing Designs." *African Journal of Reproductive Health / La Revue Africaine de la Santé Reproductive* 13, no. 4 (2009): 9–24.

Stainton, Tim. "Disability, Vulnerability and Assisted Death: Commentary on Tuffrey-Wijne, Curfs, Finlay and Hollins." *BMC Medical Ethics* 20 (2019): 1–6.

Steinberg, Laurence. "Does Recent Research on Adolescent Brain Development Inform the Mature Minor Doctrine?" *Journal of Medicine and Philosophy* 38, no. 3 (2013): 256–267.

Stinton, Sara, Barry Bogin, and Dennis O'Rourke, eds. *Human Biology: An Evolutionary and Biocultural Perspective.* Hoboken: Wiley & Sons, 2012.

Swain, James E., Jeffrey P. Lorberbaum, Samet Kose, and Lane Strathearn. "Brain Basis of Early Parent–Infant Interactions: Psychology, Physiology, and in Vivo Functional Neuroimaging Studies." *Journal of Child Psychology and Psychiatry* 48, no. 3 (2007): 262–287.

Tanz, Jason. "Playing for Time." *Wired*, January 2016. https://www.wired.com/2016/01/that-dragon-cancer/.

Tate, Tyler. "What We Talk about When We Talk about Paediatric Suffering." *Theoretical Medicine and Bioethics* 41, no. 4 (2020): 143–163.

Tate, Tyler. "Your Father's a Fighter; Your Daughter's a Vegetable: A Critical Analysis of the Use of Metaphor in Clinical Practice." *The Hastings Center Report* 50, no. 5 (2020): 20–29.

Taylor, Charles. *The Language Animal: The Full Shape of the Human Linguistic Capacity.* Cambridge: Belknap Press of Harvard University Press, 2016.

———. *Sources of the Self: The Making of the Modern Identity.* Cambridge: Harvard University Press, 1989.

Thatcher, Adrian. "Theology and Children: Towards a Theology of Childhood." *Transformation* 23, no. 4 (2006): 194–199.

Thienprayoon, Rachel, Ryan Campbell, and Naomi Winick. "Attitudes and Practices in the Bereavement Care Offered by Children's Hospitals: A Survey of the Pediatric Chaplains Network." *Journal of Death and Dying* 71, no. 1 (2015): 48–59.

———, Simon C. Lee, David Leonard, and Naomi Winick. "Hospice Care for Children With Cancer: Where Do These Children Die?" *Journal of Pediatric Hematology/Oncology* 37, no. 5 (2015): 373–377.

Tolkien, J.R.R. *The Two Towers.* London: HarperCollins, 2002.

Turner, Susan M., and Gareth B. Matthews, eds. *The Philosopher's Child: Critical Essays in the Western Tradition.* Rochester: University of Rochester Press, 1998.

UK Ministry of Justice. *Assessing Risk of Harm to Children and Parents in Private Law Children Cases Final Report.* June 2020. https://tinyurl.com/378jc8m8

The United Nations on General Assembly Resolution. *The United Nations Convention on the Rights of the Child.* London: Unicef, 1989 and 1990.

Veltman, Andrea, and Mark Piper. *Autonomy, Oppression, and Gender.* New York: Oxford University Press, 2014.

Verhagen, Eduard, and Pieter J.J. Sauer. "The Groningen Protocol -Euthanasia in Severely Ill Newborns." *The New England Journal of Medicine* 352, no. 10 (2005): 959–962.

Verhey, Allen. *The Christian Art of Dying: Learning from Jesus*. Grand Rapids: Eerdmans, 2011.

Wade, Katherine. "Beyond Bioethics: A Child Rights–Based Approach to Complex Medical Decision-Making." *Perspectives in Biology and Medicine* 58, no. 3 (2015): 332–340.

Wagemans, A., H. van Schrojenstein Lantman-de Valk, I. Proot, J. Metsemakers, I. Tuffrey-Wijne, and L. Curfs. "The Factors Affecting End-of-Life Decision-Making by Physicians of Patients with Intellectual Disabilities in the Netherlands: A Qualitative Study." *Journal of Intellectual Disability Research* 57, no. 4 (2013): 380–389.

Walker, Margaret Urban. *Moral Understandings: A Feminist Study in Ethics*. 2nd ed. Oxford: Oxford University Press, 2007.

Wall, John. "Childhood Studies, Hermeneutics, and Theological Ethics." *The Journal of Religion* 86, no. 4 (2006): 523–548.

Wall, John. *Ethics in the Light of Childhood*. Washington, DC: Georgetown University Press, 2010.

Weerd, Willemien de, Donald van Tol, Marcel Albers, Pieter Sauer, and Marian Verkerk. "Suffering in Children: Opinions from Parents and Health-Care Professionals." *European Journal of Pediatrics* 174, no. 5 (2015): 589–595.

White, Michael K. *Maps of Narrative Practice*. New York: Norton, 2007.

Whytock, Carla Elizabeth. "Understanding the Self through Recognition and Mortality: MacDonald's Portrayals of Identity in his Fairy Tales for Children." *North Wind: A Journal of George MacDonald Studies* 35, no. 30 (2016): 68–88.

Wilhelms, Evan E., and Valeria F. Reyna. "Fuzzy Trace Theory and Medical Decisions by Minors: Differences in Reasoning between Adolescents and Adults." *Journal of Medicine and Philosophy* 38, no. 3 (2013): 268–282.

Williams, Bernard "The Human Prejudice." In *Philosophy as a Humanistic Discipline*. Edited by A. Moore. Princeton, NJ: Princeton University Press, 2006. 135–152.

Williamson, James T. "The Fourfold Myth of Death and Rebirth in George MacDonald's Phantastes." *North Wind: A Journal of George MacDonald Studies* 33, no. 3 (2014): 35–69.

Woo, Jeng-Chung, and Yi-Ling Lin. "Kids' Perceptions toward Children's Ward Healing Environments: A Case Study of Taiwan University Children's Hospital." *Journal of Healthcare Engineering* (2016): 1–10.

Woolley Jacqueline D. and Maliki Ghossainy. "Revisiting the Fantasy-Reality Distinction: Children as Naïve Skeptics." *Child Development* 84, no. 5 (2013): 1496–1510.

Wright, Susan. "Graphic-Narrative Play: Young Children's Authoring through Drawing and Telling." *International Journal of Education & the Arts* 8, no. 8 (2007): 1–27.

Wyatt, Kirk D., Betsy List, William B. Brinkman, Gabriela Prutsky Lopez, Noor Asi, Patricia Erwin, Zhen Wang, Juan Pablo Domecq Garces, Victor M. Montori, and Annie LeBlanc. "Shared Decision Making in Pediatrics: A Systematic Review and Meta-Analysis," *Academic Pediatrics* 15, no. 6 (2015): 573–583.

Index